WHY?

ALZHEIMER'S

Medical science and families are still asking

WHY?

Coping with shattered dreams and broken hearts, and the loss of a loved one to a frightful disease

Jim Greenwood

Alzheimer's: Medical science and families are still asking WHY?

Published by Wheatmark™
610 East Delano Street, Suite 104, Tucson, Arizona 85705 U.S.A.
www.wheatmark.com

International Standard Book Number: 1-58736-625-8 (paperback)
International Standard Book Number: 1-58736-635-5 (casebound)
Library of Congress Control Number: 2006923732

Interior design by Carol Barry Nelson
Type & Graphics

Cover design by Lori Sellstrom

To Robin Henson, whose compassion, sensitivity and tender loving care comforted Maxine and me during the darkest days of our lives.

*Nobody cares how much you know,
until they know how much you care.*

Table of Contents

INTRODUCTION

Maxine Greenwood was born Helen Maxine Gladding on October 20, 1916, in Hoopeston, Illinois. She grew up in nearby Urbana and, despite many obstacles, succeeded in fulfilling virtually every expectation, except one -- her first marriage. Though destined to fail, the union did produce three lovely daughters.

Her second marriage, to the author, was romantic and exciting for both. Yet fate often strikes without reason or favor. And the consequences can be devastating. I watched Maxine leave a world of comfort and confidence for one of anxiety and bewilderment. Instead of living for a future bright with promise, she lived only for the moment and required 24-hour care.

This is her story -- a story of a beautiful human being whose once brilliant mind became terribly confused and constrained. It's also a tale of unremitting love, devotion and faith. If in some small way it might help others who face similar challenges along life's path, then her story was worth the telling.

Jim Greenwood

CHAPTER 1

"May I have some of your time, please?"

Maxine's eyes sparkled and opened wide as she smiled broadly, that beautiful smile so familiar to so many. We were sitting in her new "home away from home," revisiting some of our more memorable experiences in happier times. She laughed almost uncontrollably as I mentioned the elegant little Swiss café where we each devoured a tasty ham sandwich that turned out to be donkey meat. Then this jovial scene vanished just as quickly as it had appeared. Life simply wasn't the same anymore.

"Why?", I kept asking myself. Suddenly I was reminded that my beloved Maxine always asked "why?" whenever she didn't understand something she was told to do. One day she refused to step into the shower. "But Maxine," said the perplexed caregiver, "you must take your shower." Max: "Why?" Caregiver: "Because Mother Nature wants you to be clean." Max: "I don't know her."

I began grieving for my precious wife long before she finally succumbed to Alzheimer's in the early morning hours of August 27, 2003. My emotional distress started in earnest on the day I placed her in a Tucson residence specializing in dementia care management. Returning home alone, it welled up inside me as I sat on the edge of an empty bed, weeping openly and muttering out loud, over and over again, "What have I done, what have I done?"

For one thing, I was immediately struck by the realization I had probably committed Maxine for the rest of her days. And for another, I felt like I had abandoned her, a feeling of guilt that has haunted me ever since. She suffered from an insidious disease for which there is no cure, nor even physical or medical means of halting or even slowing its progression very effectively.

Why?

Reverend John Ross, senior pastor of the Valley Presbyterian Church in Green Valley, Arizona, where Maxine is interred in the church's Columbarium, once told his congregation that "grief is the price we pay for love." Well, I've been paying plenty and I expect I'll continue to pay for as long as I live. Ours was a very special kind of relationship. We not only loved each other deeply, we had a mutual respect and admiration for each other very rarely seen in a society that has lost its way. For those fortunate enough to find the perfect mate, as I did, the bonds of the heart endure -- even after death.

Home care is a full-time job. It doesn't stop for trips to the bank, the grocery store or post office. The constant stress of tending a loved one leaves you exhausted, yet you are reluctant to admit you need some time off. In hopes of getting some relief, I enrolled Max in a state-licensed program for people with dementia. It's conducted by Casa de Esperanza Adult Care Center during the day, five days a week.

At the center, a skilled staff provides recreational activity, lunch, and other services. For a modest fee, I could get a few hours of free time every weekday, but it wasn't in the cards. Max was extremely unhappy there, even to the point of crying, something she seldom did. So, I gave up the idea of a respite and kept my precious at home.

Now, as I reflect on our life together, I would only cherish the many beautiful memories surrounding me, not replace them. And during my frequent visits to her dwelling in Tucson, I shared with Maxine, briefly and simply, several of our favorite anecdotes that best described an idyllic marriage. Naturally, there were times we disagreed, but we were never disagreeable.

How well I recall the day she entered my office at Learjet in Wichita, Kansas, seeking a position as my executive secretary. She worked for a Wichita law firm, but wanted something more suited to her special skills, something more challenging. She knew that I'd fired three secretaries in less than a year, but that didn't phase Maxine one bit. I asked her why she wanted to change jobs, and Max said, rather matter-of-factly, that working for lawyers was about as exciting as washing dishes.

At the close of my interview, I told Maxine she had all the necessary qualifications to meet my exacting standards, then added, "But I must warn you, our founder and president, Bill Lear, is a perfectionist, and so am I. The job can be very demanding. If you take it, it won't be easy." "Mr. Greenwood," said Maxine, "if I wanted an easy job, I'd keep the one I have now." She not only got the job, she got the boss. Five years later we were married.

Alzheimer's disease (AD), the most common form of dementia, is a progressive, degenerative disease that attacks the brain, resulting in impaired memory, thinking and behavior. It is a complex genetic and environmental ailment first recognized in 1906. Researchers, however, have only recently developed a broader knowledge of the changes in the brain and personality that characterize Alzheimer's.

Symptoms include gradual memory loss, decline in the ability to perform routine tasks, disorientation, loss of language skills, difficulty in reading and learning, and deterioration in judgment and planning. There are three basic levels of the disease -- mild, middle and late. Maxine ultimately reached the most advanced stage, but I first noticed telltale signs of dementia in the late 1980s.

Always outgoing and socially active, Max began to withdraw. She had little or no short-term memory and frequently repeated herself several times in conversations. Her habits and patterns at home changed. She'd often forget and misplace things, such as keys, jewelry and the like. And most unusual, she was no longer the self-assured Maxine we had all come to know. And her memory loss was a constant worry. Fortunately, for all who knew and loved her, she never lost her sense of humor.

In early 1990, Maxine was clinically diagnosed as having a "type of Alzheimer's dementia." I immediately set out to provide all the care she might need at home. Naturally, this meant curtailing my own activities, which I was more than willing to do. Until then, our life together had been rapturous, eventful, unforgettable. In many ways, it fit the pattern of a storybook romance.

My first heart attack in 1987, and triple bypass surgery four years later, complicated matters. By previous marriages, we each had three girls of approximately the same corresponding ages -- Yvonne, Marquita and Vivienne on Maxine's side, and Karen, Roxanne and Jeanne on mine. Happily, our six offspring came to our Green Valley home in relays, each for a week at a time, during the period of my recuperation. Actually, Roxie arrived in time for my operation and hospitalization.

Following my first heart attack on Flag Day, June 14, 1987, I teased Maxine as the possible cause of it. For years she had been nagging me to quit my regular breakfast of bacon and eggs, and eat a bowl of cold cereal with a sliced banana and some dry toast instead. So on that hot day in June, I acceded to her wishes. But before I finished the meal, I found myself in an ambulance, racing toward St. Mary's Hospital with red light and siren clearing traffic. Obviously, I said to Max, the abrupt change in my morning diet was too much of a shock for my system.

After recovering from open heart surgery performed on September 18, 1991, I assumed the role of Maxine's sole caregiver, 24/7. Not that I minded, but I had no idea how stressful it can be. Still, I became pretty good at showering, dressing and feeding my precious, though it's a miracle my cooking didn't kill us both.

As we approached the Christmas holidays in 1995, Maxine, her voice filled with fear, suddenly called me to the bathroom. She pointed to a frightening protrusion between her legs. It turned out to be uterine prolapse, a condition that really tested my mettle in more ways than one. As a temporary fix, the doctor fitted her with a "pessary," which had to be replaced every 30 days, and lubricated several times a week. Consequently, for the next 18 months, I was the resident gynecologist.

Evenutally Dr. Lisa Landy, well aware of the risks involved in anesthetizing anyone suffering from Alzheimer's elected to operate, since the pessary option had run its course. On October 18, 1997, Dr. Landy performed a "Lafort colpocleisis," a procedure less invasive than a hysterectomy. I remained with Maxine at Northwest Medical Center, thinking my presence might be comforting. Actually, Max was more scared than hurting.

The operation itself was a success, but the sedation, as we anticipated, had taken its toll. Max appeared more agitated and confused than ever. Compounding the problem, her colitis, an ailment she had endured for many years, triggered Max's spastic colon more frequently now, causing her extreme discomfort. But as soon as we came home to familiar surroundings, her anxiety faded.

The post-operative visits to the gynecologist for periodic examinations finally ended. At least one ordeal was over. Now, my full attention was concentrated on Maxine's most serious condition, her dementia. And my love for Maxine grew stronger as she grew weaker, mentally and physically.

We seldom discussed the problem, though I'm convinced she feared the worst. The most telling evidence was a newspaper story about Alzheimer's that she had clipped out and hidden in the back of a drawer in her bathroom. I found it later. Meanwhile, her disability slowly worsened. Max would wander around the house at night, as well as during the day. The *36-Hour Day* is an apt title for the book on caregiving. I know, I've been there, like thousands of others caring for loved ones who have AD.

Finally, all six daughters and my own doctors insisted that I place Maxine in a residence for people afflicted with Alzheimer's.

I always believed in the old axiom "nobody tends baby like momma," and the thought of having strangers in control of my Maxine very nearly gave me apoplexy. However, the persistent physician-family alliance finally won out simply by convincing me that with my heart disease, I was akin to a walking time bomb. And if I ever keeled over, my precious Maxine would be alone, unable to handle the exigencies of an emergency.

In the early spring of 1998, Yvonne, the eldest of my three stepdaughters, joined me in evaluating more than a dozen memory care homes in the Tucson and Green Valley areas. My criteria had three main elements: first, the professional qualifications of the staff; second, the size of the facility; and third, its ambience or pleasing homey atmosphere. Maxine, of course, was with us, but she didn't have a clue as to the purpose of our inspection tour.

We chose The Gardens at La Cholla in Tucson, which was brand new and a part of The Fountains retirement complex. The Gardens had a capacity of 17 residents in each of two separate, single-story houses -- Casa Allegra and Casa Bonita. The rooms were spacious and the whole place had friendly, comforting surroundings. What impressed us most was the lead caregiver, Robin Henson, who subsequently became The Gardens' program director.

I also consulted Dr. Jessie Pergrin, a registered nurse, and one of the founders of the Alzheimer's Association Desert Southwest Chapter, Southern Arizona Region. She confirmed that we had made a wise choice, primarily because of Robin Henson, whom she labeled as one of the best in her field. When weighing decisions of this magnitude, it always helps to obtain critical input from a highly-respected authority in the caregiving community.

Unless families have ample financial resources, the cost of 24-hour care can be a key factor. Generally, healthcare industry prices reflect local economies. But room or apartment rentals and personal service fees (mine averaged some $50,000 a year) are tax deductible. Also certain medical charges are covered by Medicare or an HMO, and state aid is available to those who can demonstrate they have no visible means of support.

For me, moving Maxine was a nightmare and I doubt if I could ever have done it alone. Fortunately, daughters Yvonne and Marquita came to help me two days before we were scheduled to admit Maxine on April 26, 1998. Except for a new bed, all personal belongings, including the other furniture from our bedroom at home, plus two of her "comfie" chairs, were in her room at The Gardens by the time we arrived late that afternoon. Even her favorite pictures had been hung on the walls of her new quarters.

The trauma of transitioning from familiar surroundings to a new environment was virtually nil as a result of putting everything in place for Max ahead of her physical move. The two girls and I stayed with Max through dinner. The next day we had lunch with her, then the girls headed for their homes in California and I drove back to mine in Green Valley, where I sat down on the bed and wept. And again, I asked myself, why?

I was devastated, a basket case. My own two failed marriages had given me three beautiful daughters, but Maxine had become the center of my universe. I walked from room to room, searching for I knew not what, all alone in our Monterey-style house filled with wonderful memories, as well as heartbreaking reminders of the many happy years we enjoyed together.

My thoughts turned to Maxine's early years in Illinois, and to her many accomplishments. As a child, she was naturally curious, inquisitive. Such innate human instincts are part of a youngster's development and tend to moderate with maturity. Not so with Maxine Greenwood, however. For her, the pursuit of knowledge was always a never-ending chase, at least until her fertile mind became muddled with disease.

At the University of Illinois, she majored in journalism, not necessarily because she liked the news profession, but more because she also knew training in a discipline shaped by the techniques of inquiry would benefit her studies in other fields. Her interests were many and varied -- art, music, literature, science, history. She also was fascinated by archaeology, astronomy, geology, and geography, especially studies of the polar regions.

A voracious reader, Max absorbed volumes of material on all the subjects that attracted her. She wrote many book reviews on topics that ranged from biographies of pioneering explorers and bold adventurers to the histories of playing cards and Chinese art. "We live to learn," she once remarked. "Whenever we stop learning, we stop living."

The second of four children, Maxine's parents christened her Helen Maxine Gladding. But she much prefered Maxine over Helen. Her given name Helen or the initial "H" appeared only on legal or other official documents. In all the years I knew Max, I never heard her called Helen, with the possible exception of someone in the IRS or in a doctor's office.

I recall that Max's high IQ surfaced early. In grade school, she purposely wrote a wrong answer on one of her papers just so she could get a red check mark like all the other kids. A "Straight A" student at Urbana High School, Max served as editor-in-chief of her class yearbook, *The Rosemary*; won a coveted DAR prize for American history; and belonged to the National Honor Society. As a class valedictorian, she was chosen to deliver the commencement address for her Class of 1934.

Due to family circumstances in the depths of a severe economic depression, Maxine literally had to earn her education. She worked for her room and board in high school, then held a full-time job at the University of Illinois Health Center to pay for her living and schooling expenses. But despite the burdens of supporting herself while carrying an extremely heavy course load, she was determined to achieve academic excellence. And she did.

Maxine received her journalism degree in 1938, graduating with "Bronze Tablet Honors," a prestigious commendation awarded only to three percent of the students who had the highest average grades in their entire class. Almost immediately she landed a job at *The Daily Dispatch* in Moline, Illinois, where she was recognized as the first woman ever hired in the display advertising department.

Now, for the first time in many years, we would no longer be living together. Thankfully, my daughter Jeanne, a registered nurse, flew in from Georgia to be with me during my first full week alone, for which I was ever so grateful. Jeanne also helped me cope with Maxine's death. She arrived the day after Maxine died and stayed with me the rest of the week. Her companionship was most comforting and eased the pain of such a disconsolate loss.

It was Jeanne who suggested I maintain a daily journal or diary for the purpose of monitoring and recording the care Maxine received at The Gardens. I began it with notes I had compiled the day we prepared her room (April 24, 1998), and ended it on the day she passed away at The Place in Tucson, five years and four months later (August 27, 2003).

My entries filled 11 Omni "Assignment Books," each measuring five by seven inches in size and containing 200 lined pages. Each page provided a day-by-day account of Maxine's eating, medication, comportment and interaction with the caregivers and other residents in her building. I also noted any departure from her normal routine, such as repeated bowel movements at night, unusual sleep interruptions, and any other physical disorders.

The record revealed moments of magic and misery, contentment and disappointment. Some days Max ate 100 percent of all three meals, other days her food intake was well below par. But my being with Max didn't seem to have much bearing on her appetite. We got her to drink at least one can of nutritional supplement a day -- Ensure or Equate. She loved the strawberry-flavored Equate, "equating" it to a strawberry milkshake.

I'm certain Maxine's eating habits largely hinged on whether she was bothered by stomach cramps at mealtime, a direct result of her colitis. In rereading my entries, I noticed that she often complained of a troubled tummy during her first year of residence at The Gardens. I also noticed that she was lucid and articulate in those initial days of adjusting to her new surroundings.

At times Maxine's spirits mirrored the Maxine of yesteryear in the words she spoke and in her actions and reactions. She didn't always say my name at this juncture, but she somehow knew we were connected. And yet, if I turned from her to acknowledge some other person nearby, she might pop out with something clearly indicating her displeasure. On more than one occasion, she said, "Jim, Jim, may I have some of your time, please?"

CHAPTER 2

"Can we go to bed now?"

Alzheimer's Disease (AD) dims, then erases the short term and, ultimately, long-term memories of life's experiences. In every case it will eventually render the brain virtually useless and the victim helpless throughout its irreversible course. Occasionally, during our mornings or afternoons together at the middle stage of Maxine's disease, my reciting names, places and events might trigger a glimmer of recognition. She tried hard to respond, or at least nod her head affirmatively.

In the months and years ahead, of course, I'd see a dramatic change in her ability to express herself clearly and meaningfully. In the beginning, Maxine observed everyone she came in contact with, whether resident, caregiver or visitor. We soon came to know all the other residents in Casa Allegra, Max's house, by sight if not by name.

One of the ladies in our age group, Lucy, enjoyed the company of everyone. She was especially friendly and affectionate toward me. Lucy delighted in kissing me on the forehead or cheek as I sat next to my loved one, prompting Maxine to say, "Have you two got something going?"

Lucy was a little bundle of energy, always on the move. For a short time she was a "cause celebre" around The Gardens. She had figured out how to unlock all the doors of an always very secured building. She pulled the fire alarm. After the third time she did that, management changed the system. The fire department had warned that in the future The Gardens would be charged for each false alarm, something on the order of $1,200 per response.

Maxine was an extremely attractive woman and became even more so when her hair, worn short and stylish, turned snow white. To me she looked younger and prettier than her years. Her winning smile was infectious. It hooked me the first time we met in 1965, and in fact, captivated everyone with whom she came in contact, including Robin Henson and all the other caregivers.

I continued my outside activities with the Arizona Aerospace Foundation, Wright Flight, and Aero Club of Arizona, to name a few of the organizations to which I belonged. I also continued writing for publications and ghost-wrote numerous articles and marketing studies for the late Jim Taylor, former Learjet president.

However, nothing interfered with my devotion and attention to my precious. Much to my relief, she had given up driving about the time I had my open heart surgery in 1991, not at my request, but on her own volition. One of my most difficult problems was getting her to visit our doctor. She maintained nothing was wrong with her and we shouldn't waste our money supporting the medical profession. On those days I did get her to go, she'd enter the office and ask, "Is this the wellness clinic?"

Occasionally the doctors and I were at odds regarding Maxine's medication or treatment. In one instance I questioned the judgment of Dr. Tenney Kentro, who has an excellent reputation in the field of geriatrics and the physician I had chosen for Maxine. Unknown to me, Kentro had prescribed Xanex to calm her anxiety. Soon as I learned of it, I told him about my concerns.

Xanex made Maxine listless, lethargic. It also impaired her equilibrium. The doctor agreed to discontinue it, then prescribed a substitute -- Risperdal, a drug used to treat psychosis. It was just as bad, perhaps worse. It caused Maxine's ankles to become horribly swollen, sometimes a symptom of heart problems. Again, the doctor, confirming that Risperdal might cause swelling of the lower extremities, promptly took Max off it.

Normally, I'm not disposed to question a doctor's assessment of a patient's medical needs or treatment. But in Maxine's case, I knew precisely what she could or could not tolerate. That's one of the benefits of living together as man and wife. The same day we stopped Risperdal, I informed Max our daughter Vivienne was coming to see us. Max knew something was terribly wrong with her and she feared the worst. She said, "I hope I can make it."

Initially, caregivers thought Max was incontinent because of her frequent trips to the bathroom and repeated cases of diarrhea. I explained that Max suffered from irritable bowel syndrome, which was linked to her colitis. Her primary physician had prescribed dicyclomine, a purplish-blue capsule that offered considerable relief. (Eventually, all her pills had to be crushed and mixed with apple sauce.)

I also took issue with my primary physician, Dr. Stanley Racz, who admonished me for visiting Maxine so frequently. Obviously concerned for the well-being of all involved, he said once or twice a week was enough. He added that seeing her more often would be disruptive to Maxine, as well as to the staff, not to mention the negative emotional impact on me. "She's out of it now," said Racz, "and once or twice a week won't make any difference."

Naturally, I had no intention of following the doctor's orders. So I went to a "higher authority," Robin Henson, who by now had grown to know me about as well as she did Maxine. Robin quickly put me at ease. She said my daily visits were not in any way disrupting Maxine or the staff. Rather, they were good for Max and, indirectly, good for the staff.

I also knew my being there was having a positive effect just by her reactions to my storytelling and reading. I read the story of *Maxine Greenwood and the Little Mermaid* dozens of times. The small book is personalized. Max's name and the names of her three girls, Yvonne, Marquita, and Vivienne, are interspersed throughout the printed text. The first time I read it to her, she said, "That's silly." But the second time when I came across Marquita, Max said, "That should be 'Marquita May'." May is Marquita's middle name. Her birthday is May 1.

On every visit I tried my best to wear a cheerful face and say things that might make Max laugh, even though I'd repeat the same stories and jokes over and over again. For instance, I'd tell tales of our childhood, despite the fact we were both in our forties when we first met in 1965. Yet reminding Max of amusing incidents when she was a youngster seemed to strike a chord of comprehension. Not always, but much of the time.

"When you were a little girl," I'd say to Maxine, "you were quite mischievous. In the first grade, you talked so much the teacher taped your mouth closed. You tore it off, so the teacher sent you to the cloakroom. But you got even. You pulled all the wraps from their hooks and piled them on the floor."

The egg story also made her smile. As a child, she did not like soft eggs. One morning at breakfast, her mother, seeing that Maxine hadn't touched her eggs, said rather directly, "Now Maxine, you're going to sit there until you eat those eggs." Soon as her mother left the room, Maxine quickly and quietly dumped the eggs down the toilet. Her mother returned, saw the clean plate and said, "Now you see dear, those eggs weren't so bad, were they?"

Max also got a kick out of hearing about my days as a kid. I told her that when I came home from my first day in school, my mother asked, "Well, Jimmy, what did you learn in school today?" I said, "Not much, I gotta go back tomorrow." She almost split her sides when I mentioned what my father said after reading my high school report card: "One thing's in your favor, son. With grades like these, you couldn't possibly be cheating."

Humor worked well as a spiritual tonic, as long as I kept my jokes and stories short, simple and to the point. I was the center of her attention, no matter who else was present, including family. She tried her best to converse, but her words were becoming jumbled and, at times, incoherent. Yet if something happened or was stated affecting or implicating Max at that precise moment, she bounced a few choice words right off the wall.

A video producer contracted by the University of Arizona came to The Gardens one day to begin taping several residents for a two-part training guide on the techniques of communicating with persons having Alzheimer's. Because I had prepared a "Memory Book" filled with photos and captions highlighting our married life, Maxine and I were asked to participate. Specifically, the producer wanted to show us leafing through the pages of Max's new album.

If properly done, memory books can be the most effective means of communicating with dementia victims who are unable to recall the most significant events in their lives. The camera crew was in place at the appointed time, along with a small audience eager to watch the filmmaking. I arrived on schedule, the book under my arm, and walked toward the sofa where Maxine was sitting. She spotted me and, much to everyone's surprise, called out in a loud voice, "Can we go to bed now?"

The onlookers tried to stifle their laughter, but the remark tickled me, too. That was my precious. The staff had gotten her up early that morning so she could finish breakfast in time for the shoot. Obviously, she was already tired. And, as often occurred, she responded spontaneously with the first thought appropriate to the circumstances that came from the deep recesses of her diseased mind. Now, every time I watch the U of A video on my VCR, I recall Maxine's impulsive greeting just before the cameras rolled.

We frequently reviewed her memory book; it was always a whole new experience for Max each time. Certain images of activities and people depicted in the collection of pictures seemed to register with her. She appeared surprised to see our marriage certificate in front of the photos of our wedding. She could still read then, but reading was becoming more difficult for her. Maxine said she was glad we got married and asked if we could do it again, and would I come and live with her.

I turned the page and said, "And that's the Old Presbyterian Meeting House in Alexandria, Virginia, where we were married by the assistant minister, Samuel L. McCoy, on September 11, 1970." It was a small ceremony, but a lovely one. I added that the church was one of the most historic buildings for Christian worship in America and has been going strong ever since its founding in 1772. I also said, "George Washington himself attended services there." Maxine said, "That was nice of him."

Based on my own experience, I think it's very important that caregivers and their employers learn as much as they can about the people in their care. Understanding the nuances of AD victims will enable them to interact more productively and develop the kind of activity each individual resident can enjoy. Memory books are good sources of background information on residents with Alzheimer's.

Despite some awareness of her memory loss and several other health issues, Max retained her quick wit, positive attitude, and even disposition. But obvious changes in her physical well-being as the disease gradually consumed her were very painful to witness. As former first lady Nancy Reagan put it so well, "You get tired and frustrated because you have no control and feel so helpless. You know it's a progressive disease and that there's no place to go but down, no light at the end of the tunnel."

In 1994, Maxine read Ronald Reagan's letter to the American people in which the nation's 40th president disclosed that he had been diagnosed with Alzheimer's. As she finished reading it, I studied her face and saw no particular emotional reaction, other than to hear her say, "What a shame." Yet I'm sure Maxine was struggling to keep from me the stark realities of her own health.

There are two schools of thought on the ethics of diagnostic disclosure. One says telling a person the truth about his or her Alzheimer's-type dementia should be the usual practice. But it must be done with the utmost sensitivity and in a way that avoids unnecessary despair. The other warns that in some cultures truth telling for any serious medical diagnosis is considered a burden to the individual. Healthcare professionals have experienced many agonizing discussions with families on whether their loved ones should be told the facts or an altered version of them.

In my talks with Maxine, I rarely mentioned the disease by its name. It also upset her to discuss cognitive changes, and the fact AD cannot be cured. She found some solace in news reports that its effects can be treated. One thing

Max was unable to hide, however, was the slow erosion of her ability to type without making numerous typographical errors.

Maxine had always typed the final drafts of my manuscripts -- articles, speeches, business reports, and the like. Along the way, she did a superb job of editing my original material. Occasionally I'd pull her copy of *Stunt Flying In the Movies* from the bookcase in her abode and talk about all the work we both put into it. (It was published in 1982 by TAB Books, now a division of McGraw-Hill.) And I had insisted she share the byline with me.

I'd tell Max how much fun we had interviewing some of the principals we featured in the book, all of whom were impressed by her shining smile and radiant personality. I said it was the first complete story of the history of motion picture flying between two covers and started a whole new genre of Hollywood aviation literature. (It also won two awards from the Aviation/Space Writers Association.) And I stressed that I could never have done it without her. My comments amused her.

Thumbing through the book with Maxine prompted me to remind her that screenwriter William Goldman had spent a day with us in our apratment in Alexandria, pouring through our files on early aviation. Goldman, who won an Oscar for *Butch Cassidy and the Sundance Kid*, was doing research for his next film, *The Great Waldo Pepper*, starring Robert Redford. It's a tale of barnstorming pilots in the late 1920s and early 1930s, who made a living selling rides and performing daring stunts at county fairs.

Goldman had been referred to us by *Flying Magazine*'s editors, and admittedly knew little about the era of wingwalking, plane changing and exhibition parachute jumping. He wanted to gather as much background information as he could before he started writing. I told Max that he said we had made his job easier as he departed at day's end with two thick briefcases filled with notes. Maxine had no recollection of Goldman's visit, but asked if they had ever made the movie. I said yes, and we had seen it.

Because of my positions with Learjet and the Federal Aviation Administration (FAA) during Richard Nixon's presidency, Maxine accompanied me on business trips to Europe, Mexico, and all over the U.S. We usually flew in the company jet or an FAA aircraft, which made our trips especially pleasant. In her letters to the girls, written before the onset of Alzheimer's, Max said her longstanding dream of traveling abroad had finally come true.

Later at The Gardens, I often opened Maxine's memory book to the pages showing her posed by a sailfish hanging from a tall lifting hoist. I'd say, "That's in Acapulco and you caught it all by yourself. It was 10 feet long and weighed 187 pounds, just five pounds off the women's world record for a sailfish taken in Mexican waters, according to our captain." I'd go on to tell her that several of us had gone deep-sea fishing with her, but that she had boated the biggest fish of the day. She couldn't believe it.

Maxine also met many of the heroes and celebrities she had only read about or seen in movies and television, such as Captain Eddie Rickenbacker, Jimmy Doolittle, Neil Armstrong, and presidents Nixon and the elder George Bush. When Frank Sinatra brought Mia Farrow to the Learjet factory, Max told him Mia was very pretty and he was very lucky. "Thank you," said Sinatra, "and I agree with you on both counts."

Shortly before Maxine resigned her job at Learjet to become my wife, Danny Kaye stopped at her desk to say hello. She was a big fan of his -- and he recip-rocated. He whispered in her ear about his plans to fly a Learjet on his last fund-raising tour for UNICEF, Kaye's favorite charity. With Clay Lacy as co-pilot, Kaye hoped to hit 65 cities in five days, a 17,000-mile flight across 40 states and three Canadian provinces. But the scheduled itinerary was very formidable, to say the least. Even Danny Kaye himself had some serious doubts.

"Think of it as Walter Mitty's ultimate fantasy," Maxine told Kaye. "With his own Learjet, he can do it easily." And he did. The huge humanitarian effort raised more than $4 million for UNICEF and focused on the urgent needs of millions of deprived children in developing countries. It also proved the flexi-bility and utility of the executive jet. If Kaye had flown on the airlines, no more than 15 cities could have been visited.

James Coburn was another favorite of Maxine's. As we perused her album, I'd point to the photo of Coburn with his arm pulling her toward him. (A signed enlargement was on her wall.) I'd identify the picture, describe where it was taken and say, "I'm jealous. How can I compete with a Hollywood star?" Max would look me in the eye and smile, then take my hand and squeeze it.

CHAPTER 3

"I don't know what's what."

Reminiscing together was therapeutic for both of us, though at times I had to hold back the tears. That was hard, especially since my whole objective was to amuse Maxine. If, in the course of my visit, I could evoke a laugh or at least a smile, I'd consider my mission accomplished. Mentioning General Jimmy Doolittle or Neil Armstrong only by name didn't seem to register. But when I'd briefly explain who they were and how we met them, I could detect a hint or two of recognition.

For example, it was our privilege to host General Doolittle over a weekend in Texas in February 1985. We flew him in a Learjet from his California home to Dallas for the formal dedication of a new James H. Doolittle Library at the University of Texas-Dallas campus. I told her he was the one who led the first U.S. air raid on Tokyo early in World War II (16 B-25 bombers from the deck of the carrier Hornet, April 18, 1942). Still no reaction.

Next I related our brief conversation with Doolittle as we were about to board our Learjet for the return flight. Max asked him if he had everything. He said, "Yes, and more. I also have many fond memories." After landing at Monterey Airport where we had started from, Doolittle took Maxine's arm and said, "I thank you my dear, for your gracious hospitality."

He also gave her a bottle in a brown paper sack that read, "A Little Cheer from the Doolittles." The bottle itself was labeled, "Cheap, Red Wine." Maxine got a kick out of that. Actually, the wine was produced by Vin Ordinaire Ltd., a premium blend of varietal grapes. It is one of California's most popular wines. But having a personal gift from a great American hero left an everlasting impression on Max, the main reason we never opened the bottle.

Neil Armstrong was elected to the Gates Learjet board shortly after he became the first man to walk on the moon in 1969. We saw Neil regularly. In 1983, I told him I had fallen for an ad that, for less than 50 bucks, offered the buyer a place in the cosmos. So I ordered a star named for Maxine through the International Star Registry. Granted, it's a gimmick, yet a legitimate one. The name is retained in perpetuity in registration records at Geneva, Switzerland, and in the Library of Congress.

Anyway, I said to Neil, it'll make an interesting conversation piece. But, I added, I had no idea how to plot the location of Maxine's star on the two constellation charts I received from the registry. He came to our rescue. Within minutes she had pinpointed the precise position of the "Maxine Greenwood Star" in Leo Minor. In telling her about it, I'd say that loved ones are like stars. You don't always see them, but you always know they're there.

Maxine wore a 10-gallon hat when Jane Russell was our guest at a Citizen of the West ceremony honoring Charlie Gates, chairman of Gates Learjet, in 1987 in Denver, Colorado. I'd point to a photo of us in her memory book and say, "Boy, you sure look like Annie Oakley." Then I'd explain Annie Oakley and remind Max that we had been Jane's house guests in Montecito, California. And she'd nod her head and grin.

Maxine thought radio and television soaps were for housewives who needed some diversion while ironing. She watched a little TV at home in Green Valley, less of it as her disease progressed and attention span diminished. She enjoyed Lawrence Welk and several sitcoms, notably I Love Lucy, The Honeymooners, and Love That Bob, the latter starring Bob Cummings as bachelor-photographer Bob Collins. Max first met Cummings at Learjet in Wichita. He was a rated pilot and a good friend of Bill Lear.

Cummings, who started flying in the late 1920s, owned a Beech Super 18, which figured prominently in his TV show and in a story I wrote about him for *Flying Magazine*. Later I dissuaded him from investing in a "revolutionary" two-pace VTOL (vertical takeoff and landing) vehicle called the Sky Commuter. At his request, I had evaluated his project from every angle, technically and financially, and was convinced the aircraft, as conceived, would never fly. It didn't, and Bob saved a lot of money.

We last saw Cummings at his residence in California, a year before he died in 1990 at the age of 80. As usual, Bob monopolized the conversation, keeping Max from asking about his fifth wife, a Tennessee secretary whom he had married a few months earlier. The woman had written Bob after reading a super-market tabloid's account of his fourth divorce, proposing marriage to heal his emotional wounds. And he accepted.

The impulsive "romance" had fascinated Maxine who was anxious to know the new wife's whereabouts. (We learned later she was back in Tennessee.) Cummings continued pontificating about his career, his flying and the autobiography he hoped to publish. Suddenly, he looked at Maxine, who hadn't made a sound, and said, "You sure are a chatterbox." And with the utmost of tact, Max replied, "I can learn more listening than I can talking."

I think Max was equally impressed by the residential community where Bob Cummings lived -- bandleader Horace Heidt's Magnolia Estate Apartments in Sherman Oaks. Heidt bought the 14-acre complex in the 1940s and turned it into a home for actors, movie technicians, directors, musicians, singers, and dancers. Other residents with familiar names included Barbara Hale and Roberta Sherwood. Also residing there was Bill Ficks, a friend of ours and an agent for artists, writers, and entertainers, including Cummings.

Maxine was a prolific letter writer. In our first 20 years of marriage, she kept the girls abreast of our movements wherever we lived and worked. She once wrote, "I had read a number of stories about Hanna Reitsch (the famous German test pilot and one of the last persons to see Hitler alive), and never dreamed I'd one day get to meet her... or that I'd meet some movie stars and all that... so, you'll all probably have many surprises in store during your own lifetimes -- all of you."

The biggest surprise in my lifetime was more of a shock. It was the day in 1990 when my beloved Maxine was clinically diagnosed with Alzheimer's. Although I had already observed the telltale signs of Alzheimer's-like dementia, confirmation of the debilitating disease knocked me for a loop. Oddly, the first thing that came to mind was one of Maxine's oft-used expressions: "I don't know what's what." It was her way of masking a mental block, the severity of which would get progressively worse as time went on.

As I came to grips with my dilemma, I began formulating plans to meet the greatest challenge of my life. I accepted the fact our lifestyle, as we both knew it, had come to an end. And the time remaining for her on planet earth would forevermore be marked by slowly ascending levels of helplessness and hopelessness. All I could do under such extraordinary circumstances, besides my duties as primary caregiver, were things that might brighten her spirits and make her more comfortable.

In short, I was determined to live and relive cheery moments of our many wonderful years together for as long as my Maxine had a modicum of cognizance and comprehension. I'd tell her over and over again how much I loved her. I'd say, "You are my precious," and I could see in her eyes that she knew my feelings for her -- and what I meant by my words. And yet, the puzzling questions that kept running through my mind as I looked lovingly at her beautiful face: why did this happen to us?

During the first 18 months of her "confinement," Max would say little. She'd look at me from another lifetime and I'd smile back with all the passion I could muster. We'd stare at each other with a warmth and affection so overwhelming that I, for one, would weep. And at the end of each visit, I found it heartwrenching to leave her, especially early on, when she'd say, "Don't go, please stay..."

The day I gave her the memory book, I said, "Let's celebrate. We'll go to Tucson's finest restaurant and order a lunch fit for a queen and her king." She balked at first, but with Robin's help, I got her into the car. Much to my surprise, she pulled out the seatbelt and fastened it herself -- without my help. She hadn't done that for years. I said, "This is a special occasion, you can have anything you want to eat today. She said, "A Big Mac."

I should have known, it was her favorite sandwich. In dealing with dementia, you go along with your spouse's desires. Not that I ever tried changing Maxine's mind anyway. I might go over the options again, but I left the final choice to her. As I drove to the nearest McDonald's, Max alerted me to every stop sign, every traffic light, and every oncoming car we saw enroute. In some respects, it was like old times.

The roundtrip distance between our home in Green Valley and The Gardens in Tucson is 70 miles. But even if the distance were double or triple that or more, I'd drive it as often as possible. Visiting Max regularly was my highest priority. There were various ancillary benefits, too. I quickly learned the morning shift might not check the staff log to see how residents behaved overnight, or if there had been any changes in medication or sleeping habits. Whenever I noted something amiss, I'd speak to Robin and she'd take immediate corrective action.

As a result of my observations, I'd urge family members to frequently check the quality of care their loved one receives on a daily basis, regardless of the care home's good reputation. For example, Maxine's caregivers had been instructed not to put ice in her drinks due to her proclivity for chewing it. Once in a great while, someone would forget, leaving Maxine with another chipped tooth or two.

Dementia care is a demanding profession, unlike any other. It has wide-ranging personal service responsibilities. Unfortunately, the compensation is not commensurate with the job's varied duties. Despite their dedication and unique qualifications, caregivers are human. And like anyone else in a highly-specialized occupation, they make mistakes -- not often, but every now and then.

But most important, the professional caregiver is trained to celebrate each resident for the unique individual he or she is. No two people are alike, so the services and attention caregivers provide each resident are never exactly the same. Those residents (never call them patients) with AD have at least one thing in common, however. They're all different.

As the calendar pages flipped over at The Gardens, the normal progression of Maxine's disease became more evident each successive month. Still, the thought of entering her in a hospice program was far removed from my mind. Hospice patients are considered terminal with a life expectancy of six months or less, though some defy the odds and remain in the program longer.

Gratefully, people with Alzheimer's, unlike other terminally ill patients, do not go through "five stages of grief" as theorized by the late psychiatrist Dr. Elisabeth Kubler-Ross -- denial, anger, bargaining, depression and, finally, acceptance of eventual death. They don't know who they are or why they are where they are. They become totally dependent on others. Families of loved ones with AD or some other terminal disease will generally engage a hospice when the decision has been made to discontinue aggressive or some other type of life-prolonging treatment.

Hospice service focuses on pain and symptom control, emotional well-being, and other comfort measures. A flexible option available to those suffering from a less predictable, though relatively extreme disease, is palliative care, which carries no time restriction and can be provided to patients at any time or at any stage of illness. Palliative care patients also receive pain and symptom management, but can continue with aggressive and life-prolonging treatment at the same time.

Hospice is a separate benefit usually covered by Medicare and other insurers. Palliative care services also are normally covered by Medicare and other health plans. Both of these programs are nationwide. Later, as Maxine approached the end of her life, I would reluctantly yield to professional wisdom and sign up for hospice. When that day came, I'd quickly find that wide-ranging hospice services supplemented and augmented residence caregiving in a manner that was not intrusive but collaborative.

I also attended local Alzheimer's support groups and actively participated in a number of their worthwhile programs sponsored by the Alzheimer's Association. Support groups can be consoling and instructive. They are composed of relatives and close friends of persons suffering from advanced stages of dementia. They share common concerns about dealing with distress. Their exchange of personal experiences is both stimulating and educational.

From the outset, I concentrated on improving my abilities to communicate with my soul mate. People with AD have short attention spans, among other deficiences. Therefore, I modified my own language in order to help Max understand me. I established eye contact, used simple grammar and short sentences, and always used simple words, avoiding conversation that might be convoluted. AD impairs the victim's communicative functions and memory systems.

Maxine, however, was a master at capsulizing her inner most thoughts succinctly, pointedly and fittingly to the situation of that moment. The first time we met Lisa Jamarillo of The Fountains, she thought Max was Mae, another resident. She asked Maxine if Bob was her husband. Max said, "I might have married Bob, but Jim is my husband." Lisa then sat down between us and started speaking directly to me. Maxine glared at Lisa, grasped her arm and said very firmly, "He's mine!"

That episode recalled another, less serious time when Marquita and family were visiting us. In the middle of a conversation, Max turned to Marquita and asked, "Am I married?" Her daughter responded, "You certainly are, to Jim here. You don't want another husband, do you?" Max: "I might." Quips like that, I said to the family, seemed to flow from Maxine's lips freely and naturally -- and always sent my spirits soaring. At certain moments, Maxine's mind appeared as sharp and witty as ever.

In talking to Maxine, I always spoke in a calm tone of voice and limited the amount of information I wanted her to comprehend. I could tell if I was getting through by her facial expressions. I always injected a little levity in my remarks, usually including a few brief jokes. Until my precious was unable to articulate her own thoughts, her responses were the funniest. The caregivers who got Max up and dressed in the morning would usually ask her how she slept. Max always replied, "With my eyes closed."

"I don't know what's what."

During our first year at The Gardens, Maxine's eating habits fluctuated and, consequently, so did her weight. She was bothered with stomach cramps off and on, frequently causing her to get up as much as 12 times a night just to go to the bathroom. She'd also wander the halls, asking for me by name. A caregiver, of course, would intercept Max and return her to bed.

Robin Henson directed that there would be a variety of social and recreational activities for residents whose levels of dementia dictated the extent of their participation. They enjoyed morning exercises, musical programs, and in-house games, such as bowling, bingo, puzzles, card playing, and sing-a-longs. Maxine liked the professional pianists the best (she herself had played the piano.) On days a small band performed at the house, Maxine was never a bit hesitant in saying either "It's too loud" or "I can't hear you."

Whenever I left town on a trip, which was seldom, I'd stay in touch with Robin by phone, once or twice a day. It gave my morale a big boost to hear Robin say Maxine had asked for me. Returning home, I sometimes found Maxine more animated and lucid than usual. She'd welcome me with her arms outstretched and a beaming smile. Her first words were usually, "I'm so happy. Will you come and live with me?"

Max followed Robin around the residence like a puppy dog and "helped" her prepare snacks, which were offered twice a day. Major holidays were observed with special commemorative events -- Easter, Memorial Day, the Fourth of July, Labor Day, Thanksgiving, and the most colorfully decorated, Christmas. There also were birthday parties, ice cream socials, and outdoor barbeques.

On September 11, 1998, our 28th wedding anniversary, I arrived at The Gardens early. The staff had posted "Happy 28th" on the dining room bulletin board. Maxine saw it, turned to me and asked, "What do you know about this?" I said I was just as surprised as she, but thought we should go out for hamburgers and a hot fudge sundae to celebrate our 28 years of marriage.

We returned to The Gardens a couple of hours later only to find that Robin and her staff had prepared a surprise anniversary party for us, complete with ice cream cake, balloons, and assorted goodies. Naturally, we partook of the desserts, despite our full tummies. In this instance, it appeared Max had considerably more capacity than me. I was stuffed.

Although she didn't show it outwardly, I believe Maxine knew that the staff had gone above and beyond the call of duty in their efforts to salute us on our wedding anniversary. As I was leaving late that afternoon, I introduced Max to Christine, one of the new caregivers who had helped arrange the festivities.

Why?

It was always interesting to see Maxine's reaction to someone she'd meet for the first time, whether a member of the staff, a resident, or an outsider.

Usually, Max merely exchanged pleasantries with the newcomer who, at least to her, was a total stranger. The chemistry between Max and the staff and residents where she lived was generally positive. But on occasion she'd balk at being told what to do. When I presented Christine, whom she hadn't met formally, Maxine studied her for a moment, then said, rather firmly, "And are you going to boss me around, too?"

CHAPTER 4

"Why does he have to work so much?"

In the early fall of 1998, I became increasingly concerned about the frequent swelling in Maxine's ankles. It had not been induced by medication. I'd ordered dicyclomine (purple pills) for her stomach and Nuprin for her neuralgia, but swollen extremities were something else. Max had also complained of pain under her left breast (an emergency operation in Wichita 30 years earlier had removed 30 percent of her left lung). After a complete physical examination, the doctor ordered X-rays and blood tests, all of which could be done at the residence.

Happily, the photos and tests proved negative. Walking toward Max to report the good news, she said to me, "Are you really who I think you are?" I said I was, and that the only medicines she must take on a regular basis were folic acid, B-12 and baby aspirin. And a purple pill or two for her stomach as needed. One morning, she spit out her aspirin. I said, "Max, the doctor wants you to take your morning pill, you should not spit it out." She replied rather sharply, "I didn't, it fell out."

There were times Maxine had no appetite at all and simply left everything on her plate untouched. The dietitian would then fix her a peanut butter and jelly sandwich. She could always manage to eat that, it was one of her (and my) favorites. One week she ate very well (caregivers reported her food intake by the percentage of the meal eaten), and her weight climbed back to 114. She even asked for coffee at breakfast one day, a beverage she never drank. But that morning she finished a whole cup -- and black.

Because of schedule conflicts, I arrived at different times of the day and enjoyed a meal with her as often as I could. When she eventually had problems feeding herself, I tried to be with her at mealtime to relieve a caregiver and help Max get the proper nourishment. Some days were better than others. She might say, "It's been a long time since I've seen you, what have you been doing?" Or she'd say, "I haven't seen you in a hundred years!"

In August of 1998, Robin told me The Gardens management was in the throes of restructuring and the changes could impact staffing. It was the first indication from Robin that she might be thinking of accepting another position. Her excellent reputation as a role model in the personal care industry had presented her with several opportunities for a higher-paying job at another facility. I would hate to see her depart, since she was such an important factor in my decision to place Max in The Gardens. I had always believed no one was indispensable -- until now.

It's said that love is blind. For some, perhaps, but not for me. I saw my love for Max sharply and clearly. I loved her with all my heart and soul -- and still do. In fact, the intensity of my adoration was a magnetizing force so great nothing else in life mattered much. And the power of my passionate feelings grew even greater as the shroud of Maxine's dreadful disease closed around her. Yet, how fortunate we were to have shared so many things with each other, especially our fondness for travel.

A small, pocket-size book, *Anywhere You Wander*, was Maxine's gift to me on Father's Day, June 17, 1983. It was a reminder of the fun of travel as it followed two little people packing their bags, then leaving home for a holiday and visiting some of the world's favorite places. And Maxine inscribed it: "To my love and traveling companion throughout life! Love, love, love. Max." I value the sentiment beyond words. And today, the little book rests on a table at the side of my bed.

Maxine wrote of our travels in frequent and newsy letters to the girls. Her missives chronicled our trips in more detail than anything I might have recorded. As I related earlier, my work at Learjet, and again at FAA, enabled us to travel together extensively, though to her even a business trip was a vacation. Our first big junket to Europe in 1972, involving a speech in London and an inspection tour of FAA facilities in Belgium, Germany, France, and Switzerland, plus other subsequent business obligations, was the answer to one of Maxine's lifelong wishes.

Re-reading her accounts of our journeys years ago revealed how much she enjoyed seeing new places and meeting new people. Max's words recall countless memories of a blissful period in our lives. They are uplifting, inspiring and, at the same time, saddening and humbling. For they are in such stark contrast to the changes in our lives over which we had no control. Here, then, is Max's description of her first sojourn oversees:

Dear Yvonne, Marquita, Vivienne,

In Boston, Jim attended an FAA Overview Conference (actually in Cambridge) and that morning, I went across the street to the Prudential Plaza, and looked through Lord & Taylor and other ritzy stores. In the afternoon I visited the Boston Museum of Fine Arts, which had many fine paintings, but I was lost in the maze most of my time there. By the time I found the Monets and others that I liked, it was time to return to the hotel and get our bags closed and on the way to the airport.

We were to take Pan Am, but there was a delay so we were booked on TWA for an 8:30 (or was it 8?) flight, and it didn't leave until 9:45! After the cocktail hour we were served dinner (this is now about 11:30 p.m.). At midnight the movie was shown (Black Beauty). I watched it without sound. At 2 a.m., I thought I'd get some "shut-eye" and it was dawn coming up! At 2:30 we were served orange juice -- and soon thereafter rolls and coffee! I guess it was 4 a.m. or 5 a.m. when we landed at Heathrow Airport, but there was a five-hour time difference and by the time we got to London it was about half-past noon (their time). It was fun to see Nova Scotia from the air, also Ireland, then England, and all of London spread out below us!

Jim's talk ("Hijacking and the Press") before the IATA (International Air Transport Association) PR bicentennial convention went off well. There were representatives from Japan, Australia, New Zealand, Zambia, etc., etc. I sat in on the speech and was impressed with the interest shown in the question and answer period. The group invited us to join them that evening for an Elizabethan dinner at the Great Forrester (a hunting lodge used by Henry VIII and Anne Boleyn). It was about a 45-minute ride in the country -- we went on two buses. On the way back, our bus ran out of petrol!

We were served mead (a wine made from honey), then a

sumptuous Elizabethan dinner, and were entertained by a group of amateur actors and actresses in costume singing old Eliza-bethan songs, dances, etc., accompanied by harpsichord and other period instruments.

Next day we were asked to join them on a tour, which in-cluded a boat ride on the Thames, tour of the Tower of London (where we saw the axe used to chop off heads -- gruesome -- also the Crown Jewels, beautiful), tour of the Lord Mayor's man-sion, and then lunch with the Lord Mayor of London at Painters-Stainers Hall -- really super elegant.

The afternoon bus was to include Lloyds of London, but it was by now mid-afternoon and I wanted to shop for some china flowers. So we took the "tube" back. What an experience. We had to change three times and upon arrival at Thomas Goode & Son (evidently a small branch store, not far from our hotel), it was almost closing time. Bought very little, as prices not appreciably less than here, due to the devaluation of the dollar. Then there was the problem of carrying items home -- and the store was not in the least interested in shipping them for me! (Probably because my purchase was not large.) So, I have only a small memento for each of you, which I'll bring in June -- and I could have bought the same things right here!

We took a tour of Shakespeare country -- fascinating -- and Bladon, where Sir Winston Churchill is buried. Drove past Oxford, toured Coventry Cathedral (most interesting) and next day we toured Hampton Court Palace and went to Windsor Castle, where we had a tour of the St. George Chapel. We were within walking distance of Buckingham Palace, from our hotel, but we had such a time getting through the maze -- pedestrian, subways, parks, etc. We hailed a cab in desperation. The cabbie said it's only a few hundred yards -- no need for a cab! We joined the throngs there and enjoyed that. The Queen's Band was play-ing "Georgy Girl" and "Do You Ken John Peel." We bought all kinds of literature and will now study up on what we saw. In fact, for Jim's birthday, I plan to get him This is England, *a* National Geographic *book that shows and tells about most of the things we saw and, of course, much more.*

Maxine's writing conveyed an enthusiasm for exploring new and the most drab and monotonous objects and structures, such as the look-alike, repetitive rooftops and row-houses in certain areas of metropolitan London. Of particular interest to her were the directional traffic signs uniquely British but attention-getting. For the girls, their mother's epistles are priceless keepsakes. For me, they are treasured memories of going places as a happy couple, whether by car or train, ship or plane. Here's the rest of her trip report:

London was really beautiful and clean, spring had suddenly arrived and trees, jonquils, pansies, and all kinds of flowers everywhere. Sidewalks so clean. In fact, there were "litter boxes" on street posts and if you walked your dog and he soiled the sidewalk, you had to be carrying a dustpan and little broom and clean up after him! Of course, the houses where we were (in Westminster) came right up to the sidewalks, which were quite narrow anyway. We loved the English expressions -- "flyover" was the overpass, highways were "motorways," divided high-ways were "dual carriageways." "Reduce Speed Now." "Don't Change Lanes." Yield is "Give Way." No passing is "No Over-taking." Whenever we were riding on a "Flyover," we were impressed with the sight of a myriad number of clay chimneys! And the Tudor style houses, like 111 Delrose, everywhere. But so much sameness in the houses. These we saw on the outskirts of the city and in the country on our tours. "Pay and Take" for cash and carry. You descend and ascend in the "lift."

In Brussels we were met by one of the FAA men -- such a joy! We had a marvelous lunch in a little French café on the Grand Place, then Jim spent the remainder of the day at the FAA office and I wandered around the little arcades, etc. Our hotel there was a "luxury" hotel but the least attractive of any we had. Next day a driver from the Embassy drove us to the airport. We were met at Frankfurt by one of the FAA people there and spent until 4 p.m. at the FAA facilities on Rheim-Main Air Base and I got to sit in on the briefings, which I found most interesting.

There is a brand new airport at Frankfurt and our FAA man could hardly find his way, even using a map! There were three sublevels, the lowest one is a train station. Then we flew to Paris, arriving at about 5. What a city. Busy, crowded -- cars drive on the sidewalks (that is, with the two left wheels) and park right on the sidewalk. Sidewalks are narrow anyway and walking is treacherous, they seem to be hellbent to run you down. We took a tour of Paris next day on a double-decker bus, top deck, seemed safer up there! Delightful little hotel called the Madeleine Palace, very small and quaint. We had a guided tour of the Louvre, but our guide spent too much time on Greek and Egyptian statues to suit me. Of course, we saw the Venus de Milo, Winged Victory, and Mona Lisa. She abruptly left us at the end of the tour. There were about 25 in the tour; our guide spoke with such an accent we could hardly understand her. We liked to never find our way out of the Louvre and never did find the paintings I'd have pre-ferred seeing. Only makes me appreciate the National Gallery of Art so very much more.

We spent some time at the American Embassy (where FAA's office is) and went through the Commissary; only purchased toilet paper! Perfumes were expensive, and you know how little I use. There were Christian Dior scarves for $15, etc., etc. I thought I might get a new purse, but they started at $35. This is supposed to be much cheaper than in the stores!

We called the Anselms from Paris and they insisted we come and see them and they wanted us to stay at their apartment. So Friday afternoon, being the only time we could get plane reser-vations to Geneva, we cancelled our trip to Versailles and Fontainbleu, and arrived in Geneva for the most wonderful part of our vacation! I guess having someone plan for you and who can understand spoken French really makes a difference. Harvey is with Learjet. He is manager of European operations and was at Learjet in Wichita when I started there. His secretary was Nancy Hoover, you remember her. She was fun.

Harvey remarried and his bride (as of September 29, 1970) is a darling girl (Swiss) and absolutely delightful. We en-joyed their hospitality and their lovely apartment. They took us to Montreux, through the Castle of Chillon, to Gstaad, Chamonix (France) and Yvoire. And to the most interesting restaurants where we had air-dried meat (donkey), squid, octopus, delicious vegetables, superb ice cream (glaces), and other confections, expresso, etc. Geneva itself was fascinating. And we also went through the United Nations in Geneva. All for now! Are you still awake?

Love, Mom & Jim

As I sat with Maxine in The Gardens, reviewing highlights of our first trip to Paris, I told her how she saved us a lot of money by giving our taxi drivers instructions in French. I said they're famous for taking American passengers the long way to destinations, thus hiking fares substantially. Max didn't recall knowing French, but there was a time when she could read and write the language and speak it fluently. Anyway, she appeared amused by our experiences in Europe and asked if we could go back some day.

The Anselms, Harvey and Elizabeth, had died since our visit in the spring of 1972. In reciting incidents and events to Max, I'd avoid mentioning anyone's passing. In Maxine's mind, members of her immediate family were still living. Every so often she'd ask for her mother or father, sister Jean or brother George, all of whom are deceased. On such occasions, I'd engage in therapeutic lying, as the Alzheimer's experts advise, and simply say they were home in Urbana, Illinois. News of someone's death can be extremely upsetting to persons with dementia.

I was delighted with Maxine's interest in visiting the United Nations, which succeeded the League of Nations and was actually occupying the League's buildings in Geneva, the Palais des Nations. She was aware that in 1919 President Wilson had named my father, Ernest Greenwood, the assistant secretary general and executive officer (reporting to Wilson) of the first International Labor Conference. I told her that the International Labor Organization (ILO), an arm of the League of Nations, was a product of the Treaty of Versailles. (My dad was a staunch Republican, working for a Democrat president.)

For the next three years, my dad served as the only American representative to the ILO, a post that, in effect, made him the only U.S. delegate to the League of Nations. Since the Congress never ratified U.S. membership in the League, Max thought my dad's presidential appointment was something special. She wanted to go into detail about it in her long missive to the girls, but I talked her out of it.

However, Max was just as excited as me when the public affairs officer, Terrance Davidson, invited us both to take a "sentimental journey" through the

Why?

ILO archives. The "Ernest Greenwood Papers" were all there, including Dad's reports to the president. And the papers are still utilized by students, scholars, journalists, and historians in search of official information and documentation on the birth of the International Labor Organization and its evolution down through the years.

In 1987, Max helped me compile a selection of correspondence, published articles and other material on my father's professional career, with emphasis on his many contributions toward a greater understanding of the human condition and world affairs. A prolific writer, astute political observer, and dedicated public official, he distinguished himself in the service of three presidents -- Wilson, Harding and Coolidge.

Naturally, Maxine had never met my father (he died in 1938), but she had expressed a sincere interest in knowing all about him, particularly during the Coolidge administration when he worked closely with Herbert Hoover, then Secretary of Commerce. And she shared my pride in the fact I followed in his footsteps as director of public affairs for the Federal Aviation Administration (a Nixon administration appointment). My dad had pioneered the position in 1927 when Secretary Hoover picked him to be the first information officer for the Commerce Department's new Aeronautics Branch.

The Aeronautics Branch, precursor of the FAA we know today, was authorized under the Air Commerce Act of 1926, history's first U.S. legislation designed to regulate civil aviation -- aircraft, airmen, and airports. And my dad had a role in developing certain provisions of the bill. From time to time, Maxine, always curious and inquisitive, would bring up my father's writing.

Dad authored more than a dozen nonfiction books and scores of magazine pieces on such diverse subjects as political objectives, electric power, and federal regulations. I vividly recall my father telling me, his teenage son, that if I ever intended to write or speak for public consumption, I should always use words sparingly and avoid repetition. I tried to adhere to the rule in my writing and speaking. Yet in conversing with Maxine in her impaired years, I'd use few words, of course, but usually repeated my thoughts to help her grasp their meaning more easily.

I'd also read her something I wrote and ask if I had made all the editorial changes she had suggested, pointing to several places in the manuscript, even though she hadn't actually seen the rough draft beforehand. It seemed to please Maxine that I still relied on her literary skills to polish my writing, which she had done for me so many times in the past. It gave her a sense of purpose and

-32-

direct involvement in the creative process -- and that we still functioned as a team in the pursuit of perfection and other common goals.

For much of the last quarter of 1998, Max was in fair spirits. Her eating alternated between good and not so good, and her weight, up and down. Most weeks were uneventful, but retrieving lost eyeglasses and other misplaced personal effects kept me and the staff busy searching. The first time Maxine asked me if I was her father I said, "I'm Jim, your sugar daddy." And in the days that followed, she'd suddenly say, "You're my sugar daddy, aren't you?" For some inexplicable reason, she had retained my rather innocuous statement in the deep recesses of her troubled mind.

Of course, that meant a great deal to me, even though I knew it wouldn't stick. To see her face light up whenever I arrived was worth more to me than all the gold in Fort Knox. And occasionally at bedtime, Maxine might ask for me, either by name or by a reference to "my husband" or "that man." The caregivers would always say, "He working, but he'll be back later." And invariably, Max would ask, "Why does he have to work so much?"

CHAPTER 5

"So that's how I gotcha!"

Accommodations at The Gardens were ample in size, large enough for two residents per room. Each room had a built-in divider that offered a measure of privacy for the individual resident. And the dividers contained sufficient closet space on either side. Not exactly a private home, but if equipped with the resident's own familiar furnishings, the rooms can be made cheery and comfortable. Such an arrangement can pose problems, however.

Maxine, like most AD residents, was prone to wander. More than once, Max returned from the single bathroom she shared with her roommate and climbed into the wrong bed. Special efforts were made to pair residents who had demonstrated their compatability in the same room. Yet inadvertent intrusions in the middle of the night are generally startling to the other person sound asleep.

In early November of 1998, Maxine came down with another bad cold. It got worse by Thanksgiving Day (the 26th), adding to her confusion. She even believed someone was trying to kill her. Robin explained that persons with AD who suffered from another type of ailment often experienced delusions of being attacked or harmed. After speaking with Dr. Kentro, we took Maxine to the Emergency Room at nearby Northwest Medical Center where the doctor on duty examined her almost immediately.

The ER doctor ordered an E.K.G., a battery of blood tests, and chest X-rays (to check her lungs). Next he asked Max to open her mouth wide so he could look at her throat. He smiled and said that it appeared Max had bronchitis and not pneumonia, which both Robin and I had feared at first. This was confirmed by the other tests, all of which proved negative. By mid-afternoon we were back in The Gardens, too late for the traditional turkey dinner.

The following day Max seemed to have improved, but later she became ill at dinner. She was very confused, dizzy, nauseated and unable to stand. Fearing the worst, we called 911 and paramedics arrived within minutes. They transported her by ambulance back to Northwest where I met her in the ER. The same emergency room doctor was on duty and immediately ordered another E.K.G. and CT scan. Her blood pressure was high and left eye pupil considerably larger than the right, one of several telltale signs of a mild stroke or TIA (transient ischemic attack).

A TIA, or cerebrovascular (brain blood vessel) problem, more commonly known as a mini-stroke, might be likened to a series of intermittent shorts in a car's electrical system, or a failing fuel pump might be analogous in certain recognizable ways. It results in different neurological effects, depending upon which major vessel supplies blood to which area of the brain.

Symptoms of a TIA will vary with the blood vessels involved and the brain areas they supply. If a carotid artery (a vessel channeling blood up the neck to the brain) is the culprit, the AD victim may become more confused, incur double vision and possibly have slurred speech. Though it might be an isolated episode, the individual could have more TIAs or even progress to a full stroke situation. That's why TIAs must be fully and thoroughly evaluated, the results of which may dictate possible interventions, such as new medication and/or surgery.

Confirming her TIA, the first of a number of them Max would experience the rest of her life, the doctors prescribed a carotid doppler study of her neck arteries. Naturally, the thought of any type of stroke scared the daylights out of me, but I was assured a TIA had very few lasting effects. As we were leaving the hospital, I overhead Max ask the nurse who I was. Before she responded, I caught Max winking at the nurse as if to say, "I know who he is, but does he know?"

During all these gyrations, Max had somehow injured her knee, which bled profusely. The medics patched it, but recommended she have a tetanus shot. I objected, expressing serious concerns over the possibility of a negative physical reaction. Robin agreed. She and her staff successfully treated the wound with the added assistance of a "home care nurse" we had temporarily engaged. Again, Maxine thought I was her dad. I told her I was her loving hubby. She replied, "Oh yes, of course."

Maxine's carotid doppler tests at Northwest on December 3rd frightened her, but I remained at her side, holding her hand the whole time in an effort to calm her. The tests were favorable. Sound and images showed the right neck artery was clear, the left had a 10 to 15 percent blockage. Lab technicians said not to worry. If the interference reaches 80 percent, it's time for concern.

I was greatly relieved. As I helped dress Maxine at the end of the examination, I said to her, "Okay honey, we're finished and everything's fine. You passed the test with flying colors. Let's go home." Max said, "Oh, that'll be great!" Back at the residence she acted more like her usual self, reasonably content, though in her words, "a little mixed up."

December also marked appointments with Maxine's eye doctor, Jack Aaron, who had performed her cataract surgeries, and her gynecologist, Dr. Lisa Landy. I knew both visits (on different days) would be an ordeal. To minimize any potential trauma, I made advance arrangements to have each doctor see Maxine within minutes of our arrival at his and her doorstep. Each respective examination came off without causing Max too much discomfort, since both doctors were extremely accommodating. I was moved by the fact both doctors might not ever see Maxine again.

As 1998 drew to a close, Maxine appeared more aware of her new "home" and surroundings than earlier in the year. At times, she spoke clearly and coherently. When I showed her a photo of Vivienne, taken on Vivie's 50th birthday, Max said, "She still looks sharp." I said, "Yes, and I love her mother more and more each day." Max then said, "That's a good idea; you're the only one, and the best." Another "Maxim" that popped out spontaneously, as most of them did: "I'll try to be good. If I do something wrong, correct it. Put me on the spot."

Some days were special, particularly those when Max conversed. Occasionally, she greeted me with open arms, grabbed my hand and said, "Oh, this is wonderful, let's go somewhere quiet." Sometimes she'd ask, "Are you coming to be with me tonight?" I'd say, "We're always together in our hearts, even when we're miles apart."

While I was with Maxine, my emotions spun around like pieces of fruit in a blender. I laughed when she laughed, and I felt sad when her face disclosed an inner sadness. For me, clearly the most heart-wrenching moments of my visits came as I prepared to leave. I hated to deceive her by fibbing, but I had little choice. She'd say, "Please stay with me, live with me." Usually she'd accept my "I have to go back to the office" excuse, but more often than not she'd ask, "Why?"

Maxine's appetite still concerned me, yet at this stage of her dementia, there wasn't much we could do. However, she continued to drink her supplement all by herself, believing it to be her daily strawberry milkshake. One day she said, "I just can't remember anything these days. I'm worried we should be doing something, like getting ready to go somewhere."

Shortly before Christmas, Robin called me at 9:15 p.m. to report that Maxine had fallen in her bedroom, striking her head on a small table. For the third time in two months, Max was taken by ambulance to the Northwest Emergency Room, where she was treated for a deep scalp laceration and a cut inside her mouth. And by the time I arrived at the hospital, Max had been discharged. Robin had already driven her home to The Gardens.

Christmas 1998 was pleasant, but nowhere near as festive as the ones we had celebrated in the past, prior to Alzheimer's. Yet it cheered me to see Max eat all of her Christmas dinner, and part of her neighbor's. Also, she appeared intensely interested in the new photo album I'd brought her. Then she asked where we should live, or whether we should move at all. I said all I wanted was to be with her, and that I was willing to move wherever she wanted. And Max said, "Well, maybe we should stay put for awhile."

On the last day of the year, I gave Max an inexpensive ring from K-Mart, which I'd purchased to "temporarily replace" her wedding ring. I'd told Max her wedding ring was at the jeweler's, getting its mount repaired. Actually, it was safe at home in Green Valley. Robin had caught Maxine trying to give her good ring to another resident, a rather common trait among people with dementia. They seem to develop a penchant for giving gifts with no thought of their value. Anyway, tomorrow would be the beginning of another year of trials and tribulations.

January 1, 1999, another New Year, ambled in pleasantly at The Gardens and elsewhere. Maxine was more expressive than usual. Yet my euphoria was tempered by the realization that any exhilaration she induced in me would be short-lived. While it lasted, however, I'd revel in it, my thoughts harking back to an era of our many fun times together. My mind wandered as we sat down to a sumptuous holiday dinner amid colorful decorations the staff had arranged to celebrate this annual festive occasion.

As I helped Max get seated, she looked at me rather adoringly and said in a voice loud enough for other residents to hear, "Gee, you're handsome!" I gave her a kiss and said, "Thanks, sweetheart, but I think we'd better go back to Dr. Aaron and have both of your eyes examined again." She smiled and patted my hand.

The meal was delicious and Max consumed it all. I told her I was glad to see her leave a "happy plate" as we left for her room, where once again we went over the memory book, page by page. She suddenly asked me my name. I told her, then described the first time we met. I said she'd applied for a job at Learjet and I was so impressed with her qualifications and attitude I hired her on the spot. Max said, "So that's how I gotcha!"

Even though the disease had ravished her brain cells, Maxine was still the same gracious person I married. Her personality and moods changed almost constantly. Yet my love for her was so deep and so strong that I continued to see her as the wonderful, loving wife I had wed. My heart ached every time I saw her, but she would always unknowingly -- and unwittingly -- say something, if only a few words, that rekindled my adrenalin.

Maxine's positive attitude didn't obscure the fact darker days lay ahead. I no longer harbored denial, nor did I still hope some miracle might restore at least part of her lost memory. But by now I'd improved my ability to interact meaning-fully with Max's memory impairment. I continued to refine my communication skills and make each morning or afternoon an opportunity to build her self-esteem with formal and informal reminiscence strategies. And my cardinal rule: Anything and everything must be done to preserve Maxine's dignity and comfort.

As Max herself might say, the learning process never ceases. Every day was a new adventure. One primary objective, of course, was to strengthen the rela-tionship between Maxine and me -- and the professional staff -- through a cul-ture of caring built upon mutual respect and appreciation. I encouraged caregivers to review major events in Maxine's life history -- and the life histories of other residents in their care as well.

Some knowledge about the people with whom they interact should enable them to spark multisensory functions that might stimulate at least some dor-mant powers of recall. Memory books are good sources for brief information on Alzheimer's victims and their families. All of us have but one life to live and memories are the single most important element in our personal histories. There is no substitute for a nostalgic walk in the past, for there's a great value in looking back before contemplating the future.

For sometime, our intimate life had been virtually non-existent. Yet there were times we seemed closer than ever, rare occasions that kept me pumped up, and very possibly Maxine as well. I often sensed she was aware of our deep mutual affection. It almost erased the fact our long, joyful and adoring union had, for some mysterious reason, taken an unwelcomed detour.

By now, though, I unwillingly admitted that a single caregiver, including myself, cannot tend an Alzheimer's patient alone. The job is too big, and more complex than anyone can conceive. It's not a question of love, nor does it mean there's an absence of commitment. Simply put, it has to do with professionalism. And in the world of Alzheimer's, spouses who struggle with the caring of loved ones are rank amateurs. Anyone with stage three Alzheimer's requires a team of practical, certified professional caregivers, beginning with the neurologist and continuing with nurses' aides around the clock.

As the weeks passed, Maxine would ask for me, not always by my name, but by "my husband" or "that man," which gave me some measure of encouragement. I continued monitoring her eating habits, comfort, weight, and attitude. Her appetite varied, usually the result of sporadic cramps or a sore tooth. Her participaton in scheduled activities also fluctuated. When engaged in some sort of game she disliked, she would quit and say, "This is ridiculous."

As I looked around the room at Max and the other residents, I thought to myself that she was right in her assessment of the whole scene. It was preposterous, ludicrous. Adults, most of them in the prime of their lives, were now slowly and cruelly being robbed of their mental faculties. They had become totally dependent on others.

Time and again I asked myself why? No wonder my grieving began the moment I left my precious in the company of strangers. Grief, as a general rule, is associated with bereavement. But regardless of the circumstances, it must be authentic. Each individual must grieve in his or her own way and time. Yet it is absolutely necessary for anyone emotionally distressed to make choices and move forward. As long as extreme sorrow persists, it can be oppressive, onerous, and hazardous to one's health.

Loss is part of the mosaic of life, but growth is possible and can lead to greater promise. How easy it is to drown in the depths of deep depression. Caring for Maxine, of course, was my all-consuming project. Yet I continued to involve myself in work related to my specialized vocation in the aerospace industry, much of it as a volunteer. As my good friend Bob Serling said, "If Greenwood had been born a woman, he'd be pregnant every nine months because he never learned to say 'no'."

I didn't believe I'd ever hyperventilate, but it has occurred in the midst of a critical -- at least in my view -- assignment having a near impossible deadline. Coupled with the complexities of Maxine's care, these extraneous activities may have caused a level of stress that heretofore I had astutely tried to avoid.

Whatever I had going on, I managed to find some sort of balance toward the preservation of my sanity.

I also made every effort to keep my most significant memories tucked away in a brain cell somewhere, which I could call upon in a crucial moment. Memories are excellent reminders of the really important things worth thinking, and even worrying about. I had to put my extracurricular commitments in proper perspective.

Pressure strains both mind and body. So I told myself, why not take a deep breath and reassess my priorities. In short, exercise better control over my daily routine.

My regular visits with Maxine were a mixture of sadness and gladness -- sad to see her so functionally impaired, but glad to see her laugh at my jokes and anecdotes. Actually, her spontaneous retorts were gems. Returning from Casas Adobes Optical, where we had eyeglasses fixed for the the umpteenth time, I said, "Well, Sweetheart, that didn't take long." Max: "It's not over yet."

Maxine remained alert and conversant during much of 1999, even though I detected some slight deterioration in her speech. Several things happened that were somewhat disturbing. Once again, the doctor prescribed Tylenol, for no particular reason in my judgment. After consulting with Robin Henson, I nixed the treatment, since Max had no outward signs of any physical pain. Extra Strength Tylenol, containing acetaminophen, had caused Maxine considerable discomfort in the past. The doctor accepted my decision.

One of the caregivers, Marjorie, discovered that I'd performed exhibition parachute jumps in the days leading up to World War II. She asked Maxine, "Did you ever jump with a parachute?" Max said, "No, and I don't intend to." I changed the subject and said, "Can I have dinner with you?" Max said, "I'll think about it." I said, "You'll make me the happiest man in the world." Max: "Really?" I said, "I hate to be away from you." And she said, "That's my thought, too."

On January 18 we lost a good friend and neighbor in Green Valley, Charles "Buck" Rowe, who had died sometime during the night at the age of 102. I found his body after being informed by the "Telecare Service" that Buck failed to answer his morning call. Naturally, I made no mention of Buck's passing when I saw Maxine later that same day. Talk of death can be extremely disturbing to anyone with Alzheimer's.

I showed Max a photo taken of her, Buck, and Yvonne, her oldest daughter, some years earlier. I reminded Max how much we enjoyed Buck's company and the exciting stories of his long life, much of it spent in aviation. Though he was over 20 years my senior, Rowe and I had a lot in common and many mutual friends. He was a Naval Aviator in World War I, then became one of history's first flight examiners for the old Department of Commerce. He finished his long professional career as the southwest marketing manager for Gulf Oil's aviation products division.

Buck regaled us with tales of bombing German submarines off the coast of France, and of trying to enforce new Federal laws requiring civilian aviators (and airports and aircraft) to qualify for a license. One seasoned veteran pilot refused to undergo the regimen for Federal certification. "Hell," the flier told Rowe, "I have more time in forced landings than you have in the air."

The metaphor puzzled Max, so I explained that up until 1926, all civil aviation in the U.S. was unregulated. Anyone could legally fly any kind of machine without a license provided he or she could get it off the ground. However, Maxine gave a hint of recognition when I told her of the difficulties Buck was having with one of his neighbors who kept complaining about his new set of dentures. To shut him up, Buck, who also wore new false teeth, said, "Hell, I'm having a hard time chewing hard liquor."

CHAPTER 6

"Did you make that up about me?"

Residents of nursing homes, assisted living establishments and other facilities delivering personal services are exposed to a wide variety of contagious maladies. Every effort is made to sanitize each place, but it is nigh impossible to thoroughly sterilize the air we breathe, even in a confined space. Maxine was given annual flu vaccines, yet she suffered her share of colds and other viruses. Among the elderly, there is always an inherent danger of having a congestive respiratory problem develop into an inflammation of the lungs -- bacterial pneumonia or worse, viral pneumonia.

Fortunately, both Maxine and MiMi, her roommate at The Gardens, had effective immune systems that warded off many of the bugs. A lovely lady, MiMi (her given name was Hazel), ignored me as I escorted Maxine to the bathroom they shared and helped her potty. At times, Max's lower intestine became impacted and I'd summon Robin to my aid. Robin had a special technique for clearing blocked colons and voiding the alimentary canal (bowels) at the anus.

Every room was equipped with at least two buttons or cords to activate the house intercom in case of an emergency or some other need for assistance. Trouble is, most of the residents were so far advanced in the state of their disability that finding the button to push, or cord to pull, was virtually impossible. Maxine was no exception. But at least she could still find the bathroom alone during the first two years of her residency.

At the outset, Maxine's brother Don Gladding and his wife Nell, and daughters Yvonne, Marquita and Vivienne, visited with some regularity. Visits by my biological daughters, Roxie, Jeanne and Karen, were less frequent, but they were welcomed just as warmly. Usually the girls and Don brought some sort of gift, such as candy, flowers or wearing apparel. It soon became obvious that "one-on-one" visits were best. More than one person talking to Max at the same time proved to be confusing. She simply couldn't follow or understand the conversation and became frustrated.

I'd recommend that visitations to anyone with dementia in a care home be limited to one or two persons in order to maximize the quality of your time together. For example, several of us tried to persuade Max to attend a cosmetics program in Casa Bonita next door. But our urging met with strong resistance. We got as far as the outside gate when Max decided she'd rather "go home." We got back just as a caregiver declared Maxine's missing eyeglasses had been found, news that made everything right again.

Here's another suggestion for those close to a victim of AD. Write your own memoirs. It'll make it easier for you to compile that essential "memory book" for your loved one. In fact, it will serve two purposes. It'll give you something to talk about during your visits. And equally important, such a personal account of your own life can be meaningful to your descendents, as well as to the relative or friend afflicted with the disease.

No, I'm not suggesting you aim for the "best seller" list, or even the local newspaper. Writing is hard, even crazy, but it can be uplifting. A word of caution: Don't leave the material in your computer. Unless your story is transformed into hard copy, it can be lost forever. And that would be tragic.

What inspires writers? In his book *American Writers at Home*, author J.D. McClatchy writes that Herman Melville's inspiration for *Moby Dick* came while gazing out the window of his study. The hills outside had two small summits that resembled the hump of a sperm whale's back. William Faulkner wrote out plot lines in pencil on his bedroom walls. Ernest Hemingway got going by sharpening 20 pencils and Mark Twain warmed up to writing by playing billiards. The nonprofessionals, however, should just sit down and write what stands out in their lives. My inspiration: Maxine.

Julie Andrews, star of stage and screen and one of Maxine's favorites, turned to writing after a near disastrous operation on her vocal chords. And she is just one of thousands whose unique experiences and traditional values are worth passing on to coming generations. Unable to sing as before, Andrews overcame her total despondency by writing -- not only her memoirs, but a whole series of books for children.

Max and I never had any direct contact with Julie Andrews, but we did meet her talented husband, producer-director Blake Edwards, creator of the Pink Panther movies. And I did some work for one of Blake's associates, Ken Wales. I served as Ken's technical advisor on several feature-length films -- Blue Yonder, The Aviator (the original about flying the mail in the early days), and Squadron 101, which never got beyond the conceptual stage. It was fun to reminisce with Max about our Hollywood connections.

Interestingly, early in 2004, the National Endowment for the Arts asked U.S. soldiers and their families to write down what they saw, felt, and heard during the Iraqi War for a program to be called Operation Homecoming. Thousands of reflections of how military men and women react to combat were compiled in a unique documentary. They offered a cogent first-person account of the most dangerous side of service life. The troops soon learned that writing down their experiences was excellent therapy and good for the soul.

Maxine was a fine writer herself. A meticulous researcher, she had imagination, intuition, industry. I once mentioned William Faulkner's precept on being a writer: "Read, read, read. Read everything -- trash, classics, good and bad, and see how they do it. Just like a carpenter who works as an apprentice and studies the master..." (Faulkner's 1935 novel *Pylon* was the result of his keen interest in closed-course air racing.)

An avid reader, Max wrote book reviews for publication, but she'd much rather edit than write. She excelled as an editor and agreed with my favorite description of writing. It's 15 percent inspiration, 25 percent perspiration, and 60 percent exasperation. Nevertheless, I encouraged Max to take pen or typewriter in hand and commit her own fascinating life story to paper. Unassuming and modest to a fault, she saw little worth in doing it, despite all the reasons already mentioned. She tended to minimize her impressive achievements against near impossible odds.

Shortly before retiring in 1985, I suggested we might consider establishing a creative writing service that catered to businessmen who needed help with their written communications -- letters, sales presentations, marketing studies, Internet research, even web site content. Like many good ideas, it crashed under the weight of more immediate priorities.

As the reader must know by now, I follow AD research closely. Of special interest in recent years were University of Chicago studies indicating mentally and physically active people tend to have less Alzheimer's disease. They revealed that education and exercise "supercharge" a broad set of genes involved in building a healthier brain. Other scientists have also reported that genes can become activated with exercise.

Genes are involved in maintaining the health of neurons, constructing syn-optic connections between them as new memories are laid down, and building arterial highways to supply more blood and nutrients to the brain. Additional research may lead to finding exactly how mental and physical exercise pro-moted enhanced actitivity of key brain genes. The research supports a growing belief that prevention strategies rooted in exercise and education may work.

As one of the top students in her University of Illinois class of 1938, Maxine continued to soak up knowledge until the impact of AD pillaged her mind. Though she kept her brain and body active, it obviously wasn't enough to resist the onset of Alzheimer's. With reference to the Chicago study, it was also noted that broad epidemiological observations about education and exercise were, in fact, related to a reduction in Alzheimer's disease.

Consequently, if the level of physical and mental activity continues to de-cline in our population, a major issue in today's placid society, the AD epidemic may grow at an alarming pace. In other research, however, scientists found that patients with AD who were given gene therapy seemed to regrow damaged brain cells and experience a slower loss of their ability to think and remember. Yet the trial therapy was not without danger. Two patients who were treated while conscious but sedated, suffered brain damage when they moved during the procedure.

For this gene therapy experiment, researchers took skin cells from eight patients with mild AD. They genetically modified the cells to produce a sub-stance called nerve growth factor, or NGF, a protein that prevents cell death and stimulates cell function. Next they infused these genetically engineered cells back into the patients' brains. If validated in further clinical tests, this may represent a substantially more effective therapy than the current treatments using already approved medications.

During the nearly five and half years Maxine resided in a care home, I was given several opportunities for her participation in Alzheimer's research pro-grams -- clinical studies well funded, well established, and highly recommended. However, I declined each overture. After consulting specialists in the field, I felt the risks to Maxine's health were simply too great. Besides, she was in the "late" stage of AD, the most advanced of the three levels of the disease. But as long as I live, I'll continue to support AD research in other ways. It's woefully underfinanced.

Maxine had long been a student of language, which indeed made her a superb editor. Even at the peak of her illness, her words of endearment came right out of the blue, usually as a part of some distant thought process. Once, after we had embraced and kissed, Max abruptly said, "Let's get going and do what we're supposed to do, whatever that is." Caregiver Maria, standing nearby, said to Max, "You sure have a nice husband." Maxine looked Maria straight in the eye and said, "I know that!"

As time passed, Maxine was alternately in good spirits and dejected. Much of these contrasts in her comportment I attributed to her stomach problems. Her purple pills (dicyclomine) gave her some relief, but not always. Even with her discomfort, however, she never turned down ice cream or cheese crackers. She'd wash them down with a glass of her 350-calorie supplement. Max drank slowly, but once said, "Wish I could take a big swig, then I'd be ready for anything."

She probably ate more peanut butter and jelly sandwiches than anyone else in The Gardens. It was the preferred substitute for anything and everything she might refuse on the regular menu. Some other foods she especially enjoyed included egg salad, chicken salad, orange wedges, and all kinds of custard -- mostly things easy to chew. Her teeth were becoming a problem.

My spirits rose and fell with Maxine's changing emotions. And images of the many good times we had flashed through my brain like a kaleidoscope run wild. Because of Maxine's positive reactions, I delighted in painting word pictures of the motor trips we took when we were still living in the east. The felicity of language has always been a powerful tool in winning hearts and minds. Once in a while, my verbal syntax would derail, but Max seemed to revel in my short descriptions of our touring together.

One journey was especially enjoyable. We departed on her 56th birthday, headed for Briarcliff Manor, New York, where I had lived in the 1930s, and on through New England all the way to Provincetown at the end of Cape Cod. I struggled to recall certain details which had impressed her the most, but back then her memory was far better than mine. She spoke eloquently of this particular junket in a letter to the girls written the day after we got back. Here's a portion of the text in her words:

> We left about 1:30 on Friday, my birthday, and crossed the Tappan Zee Bridge at sundown, and could see the lights of George Washington Bridge and the silhouette of Manhattan's skyscrapers. We made a sharp right off the parkway onto Route 9 and were in Tarrytown (home of Rip Van Winkle, the legend of

Sleepy Hollow, etc.). We passed up the only two motels, then drove on a "spooky" road to Briarcliff Manor, where Jim went to high school, and drove around the sleepy little village.

We finally found a motel on the Sawmill River Road, and the next morning returned to Briarcliff in the daytime. We looked up C.B. Colby, who inspired Jim to write and illustrate (did you know Jim did newspaper cartoons at one time?). He and his wife were delightful. He has written his 100th book and in 1962 his copies reached one million. He writes for children in the 8 to 14 age group. You may have some of them in your libraries, for they are very popular. He wrote one on the FBI and it was this contact that inspired the naming of Erskine's buddy as Colby (on TV's "The FBI"). On our return, we had a letter from him, telling us how much he enjoyed our visit.

I must interrupt to relate an amusing story about a young boy who asked a librarian if she had any "dirty" books. The question shocked her so much she had trouble regaining her composure. But further discussion with the youngster disclosed that what he wanted was one of the C.B. Colby books. The little volumes were in such demand they were becoming threadbare and soiled -- all the marks of constant use, hence the dirty book appellation. Colby's series for Coward-McCann covered the more exciting professions: What it's like to be a policeman, fireman, pilot, etc. Here's more:

Jim also knows the Burns family, who started the Burns Detective Agency and we went to their offices (their international headquarters), and learned that his friend was in the hospital with an infected toe, which he hurt playing golf! The house where Jim's family lived has been replaced with a church; the rest of the little village remains much the same. We also drove through Pleasantville (very close) where Jim worked at Reader's Digest *after high school and saw their new facilities (from the road only) in Chappaqua, NY. We arrived at Roxie's late in the afternoon Saturday. They are close to Worcester, Mass. Boston is somewhat farther, but it seems no one goes to Boston unless they have to. The way Easterners drive, I think it wise. They pull right out onto the highway without ever looking! Shannon is a darling and took to us right away. She is walking, but not steadily as yet. She is the happiest baby I've ever known. She'll be a year old in November.* (Author's note: Shannon was the first of Roxanne's two daughters, both now grown with their own families.) *We left Shannon with her daddy Sunday and went to visit Sturbridge Village, which is something like Williamsburg, only more of a country-type village. They had a huge crowd. It is only about 30 miles from Northboro, where Roxie lives. We watched them make pewter spoons, make designs for copies of antique chairs, etc. This is the 25th year of its existence, and they call it a museum of rural New England life.*

We left Tuesday morning and drove to Quincy, Mass., where I planned to go through John Adams' and John Quincy Adams' homes, but they were closed for the season. So we took a snapshot of the outside. (I was inside the houses in 1964, but wanted to see them again. I am reading Those Who Love, *by Irving Stone, about John and Abigail Adams.) We then drove to Cape Cod, to Provincetown. We stayed at a motel overlooking Cape Cod Bay.*

We watched the fishermen bringing in their catch to the pier, and we also went to the Pilgrim Monument and the museum, which is one of the most fascinating museums I've ever seen. They had an especially interesting "Mayflower Room" which had a replica of the Mayflower, and several dioramas depicting the landing of the Pilgrims, the first wash day, the first encounter with the Indians, the finding of a spring (water). I am sending a booklet to Marquita (please share with Viv) which may give you some ideas for a Thanksgiving unit or storytelling for your classes.

Maxine and I also stood at the marker where the Pilgrims first came ashore at Provincetown (not Plymouth Rock). Years later I became aware of my astonishing link with English history. Several members of my extended family were into geneology and sent me some information about one of our more celebrated ancestors, John Greenwood (1556-1593). It appears John's advocacy for the separation of church and state so ired Queen Elizabeth that she had him jailed for seven years -- then hanged.

John and a co-worker, Henry Barrows, who was also executed for his beliefs, founded the religious doctrine known as Puritanism, which led to the English Civil War, or Puritan Revolution, and the establishment of Presbyterianism under Oliver Cromwell. The little band of Pilgrims who fled from religious persecution in England in 1620 included John Greenwood's followers. And his teachings, the right to worship according to the dictates of the individual's own conscience, formed a cornerstone of the American constitution. But Maxine's missive continues:

> *We left on Thursday and arrived too late to see anything of Mystic Seaport that eve, but we went over to New London to the Coast Guard Academy and went aboard the Eagle. We had a grand dinner at the Seamen's Inn in Mystic, then on Friday we spent most of the day at Mystic Seaport. We really enjoyed every minute of it and I believe we were in every building. We left about 3 o'clock and drove to Hartsdale, N.Y., where we looked up the cemetery where Jim's mother and father are buried. But it was closed. We drove on, in the rush hour, and by the time we reached the end of the New Jersey Turnpike Jim was numb and I was glad to stay overnight in New Castle, Del., where William Penn landed. Saturday we came home in rain and fog, but arrived at noon... our car (a sporty-looking 1965 Mercury Cougar) worked fine all during the trip -- except once our horn wouldn't work and we got rather panicky. We soon found a mechanic to connect the right wires again. In New England, you need a horn!*

Having access to Maxine's many letters refreshed my own memory as I reconstructed for her the prominent features of our numerous business and holiday travels. Actually, her own words reviewed the specifics best. A model of brevity, she "used words sparingly and avoided repetition." For one thing, she recorded her impressions immediately. For another, the documentation served us both well in the closing years of our lives together.

As I told and re-told stories of the fun times, Max's animated reactions convinced me that much of what I said got through. When I'd gaze at my precious adoringly, the sentimental side of my nature rose to the surface like bubbles in a bathtub. Martin Luther (1483-1546), the German reformation leader, once said this: "There is no more lovely, friendly and charming relationship, communion or company than a good marriage." I read the quotation many years after I wrote the following verse, which says how I felt about my beloved Max:

Of all the things that we have done,
the people and places we have seen;
My heart tells me there is only one,
the love of my life, my own Maxine.

When I recited my little poem to Max the first time, she studied my face rather incredulously and asked, "Did you make that up about me?" I said, "I'm guilty. I'm no poet, but those words came to me almost as if they'd been engraved inside my head forever. It's just the way I feel. Do you like it?" Maxine: "It's beautiful. Please say it again."

CHAPTER 7

"All this for me, why?"

The first question I asked when Maxine was formally diagnosed with Alzheimer's disease: "What can I expect?" It's a very tough question. An even more difficult one to answer is: "Why?" Then later I learned a scientific study suggested that assessing several key clinical aspects of the disease soon after it had been verified might help families and physicians better forecast the long-term survival of persons with AD.

For example, a study funded by the National Institute on Aging (NIA) and National Institute of Health (NIH) provided insights that could help public health officers refine cost projections and plan personal services for the growing number of older Americans at risk of AD. Researchers found that in the years following diagnosis, people with AD survived about half as long as those of similar age in the U.S. population. According to their findings, women tended to live longer than men after diagnosis, surviving about six years compared to men who lived about four years.

However, the gender gap narrows with age. Age at diagnosis is also a factor. Maxine was 74 when diagnosed by a doctor. Persons in their 70s are expected to have longer survival times than those diagnosed at age 85 and older. Maxine lived for another 13 years after diagnosis.

For doctors, evaluation data can be very useful for gauging the prognosis of an AD patient. And for caregivers, it can help in making appropriate plans for the future. In some respects, I'm glad no survivable data on estimated longevity was available when doctors confirmed Maxine's symptoms. I assiduously tried to avoid the inevitable. The thought of Max leaving me was almost too much for me to bear.

Yet, as a pragmatist, I knew the advantage of having some clear vision of what lay ahead. I realized Maxine's dreadful disease was an irreversible disorder of the brain. It had already robbed her of her memory, and eventually would steal her mental and physical functions as well, leading to her demise.

In fact, clinicians predict that the risk of death from AD will increase up to 66 percent during the first year following its diagnosis. Walking problems, congestive heart failure, frequent falls, diabetes, and ischemic heart disease are other indicators of reduced life expectancy. At this writing, it is computed that 4.5 million people currently have AD, and the number will double every five years after the age of 85.

For obvious reasons, I tried to learn as much as I could about Maxine's anticipated longevity. There were several things on my agenda while she possessed even a modicum of understanding. One of the most important, to me at least, was the creation of a memorial in her honor before the disease obliterated all rationality. This had long been a fervent desire of mine. And one day early in 1999, I realized I'd better get with it when Max said, "I'm looking at you, but you don't look like you."

Alzheimer's had already stifled Maxine's memory, but uniquely, she still responded to even a casual mention of the University of Illinois. She never boasted of her academic record there, but I knew that inwardly she was mighty proud of it, and rightly so. That's precisely why I chose the U of I as beneficiary of my salute to Maxine. I contacted the University of Illinois Foundation and got the ball rolling. Within a few weeks Bernie Freeman, director of the U of I Foundation's Presidents Council, and Jeff Roley, a trust officer, were meeting with me in the office of my attorney, Tim Olcott.

I'd proposed substantial cash gifts to the University's College of Communications that would fund (1) a much-needed classroom for broadcast journalism students, and (2) an endowment for scholarships, fellowships, and teaching awards, both in Maxine's name. The new classroom would be known as The H. Maxine Gladding Greenwood Video Editing Suite. The endowed tribute would be called the Maxine Gladding Greenwood Award. Both would honor Maxine's memory in perpetuity, or for the life of the university.

We drove to The Gardens where Bernie and Jeff met Maxine for the first time and promptly fell in love with her. When we entered the foyer, Robin Henson called out to Max and said, "Jim's here!" Maxine said, "It's about time." Bernie gave her an official U of I citation testifying to her academic and professional achievements. After Jeff read it to her, Max looked directly at Bernie and said, "Want to touch me?" It was a magic moment.

Clearly, Maxine was struck by all the adulation. While Max's modesty and humility smothered her pride, you could easily tell she was pleased by the flattering accolades recognizing her outstanding accomplishments under extremely difficult economic circumstances. She turned to me and said, "All this for me, why?" And I replied, "Because of the fine example you set for the rest of us, but more because I love you so much."

Nothing I've ever done in my personal life has ever given me more satisfaction than honoring my beloved Maxine at her alma mater, the University of Illinois. Due to the size of my gifts, Max and I were conferred life memberships in the University's Presidents Council. In the following months, I worked closely with the late Kim Rotzoll, dean of the U of I's College of Communications whose untimely death in 2003, on the eve of his retirement, was a tremendous blow to all who knew him. A finer man I've never met.

After our guests from Illinois departed that day, I drove to Columbus, New Mexico, where I had been doing some research on the infamous raid by Pancho Villa's guerrillas in 1916. When I told Max about the savage attack on the little town, she immediately said, "I remember, that was the year I was 'borned'."

Max then added, "I'm glad you're here, we've got to get away from all these dumb dumbs." She pointed to one of the residents and said, "See, there's one of them now." Such derogatory comments were strictly out of character, but with AD, impromptu remarks are the norm. Maxine also told Kimberly, another caregiver she liked, that I thought she was "taking up with another man," and that other people were lying about her. She said, "I'm afraid of what my husband might think."

Kim tried to convince her not to worry, that "Jim knows you love him, and only him." Max didn't bring it up again, but during a subsequent visit, she again asked me, "Are you my daddy?" As we rested on her bed, she kept repeating "I love you" which pumped me up the size of a barrage balloon. Caregiver Christine dropped by the room prompting Max to say, "I'm not your boss, you can do anything you want."

Every so often I'd pause to take stock of my performance as a caregiver, even though Maxine was now in the care of professionals. No one taught me how to interact with someone suffering from memory loss. Dealing with dementia victims is usually counter-intuitive. In other words, the right thing to do is frequently the opposite of what my intuition tells me is the correct thing.

For instance, if Max acted in ways that made no sense at all, I might be inclined to carefully explain the situation, calling on her faculties to perceive the appropriateness of a contemplated act. But persons with AD no longer have judgment cells in their brains. Consequently, they don't respond to our recommendations, no matter how logical. Short, simple sentences addressing what's going to happen next are generally best. If someone wants to go home, say, reassuring them they are home can trigger an argument. Redirecting the individual can produce an aura of calm.

There's no such thing as a perfect parent, nor is there a perfect caregiver. Caregivers, myself included, have a full range of human emotions and reactions. At times we become frustrated and impatient. I once asked an authority of Alzheimer's to list three things he considered to be foremost in the basic criteria for good caregiving. He said, "Patience, patience, patience."

Maxine had instances of lucidity. Talking with her, I had to remember I was responding to a complicated disease and not to the person she once was. And I didn't dare to imagine she was perfectly normal when she had one of those moments to be treasured. One afternoon she greeted me saying, "I'm happy to see you. I must tell you about the awful things I've been doing." (Actually she had spilled juice all over the front of her blouse.) The same day I was particularly heartened by the following exchange:

"You are my precious," I said to Maxine. Max: "If that's so, we'd better do something about it. I love you, I love you lots." I said, "I belong to you, and you belong to me. We belong to each other." Max: "That makes a lot of excitement for me." I said, "Sweetheart, I worship you and I've got you on a pedestal higher than an elephant's eye." Max: "I hope I don't mess it up."

I've always been meticulously honest with people, especially with my wife. However, after Maxine developed dementia, I soon realized honesty in some situations could lead to distress for both of us. As a result, I practiced "therapeutic lying" months before I moved her into The Gardens. It didn't matter if Max thought we were going to the store, and on the way stopped to see her doctor. Nor did it matter if I told her the lady from the family assistance center was a neighbor who had dropped in to keep her company while I attended an important meeting.

I never put a spin on stories about the University of Illinois and my plans for a permanent memorial in her honor. One afternoon I showed her the photos we were considering for the bronze plaque to be hung on the wall of "her classroom." Max studied the pictures, then pointed to one of them and said, "It looks better than I really am." Pointing to another, she said, "It doesn't look like me, but they did a good job, I like it."

Maxine, unlike most of the other residents, was rarely out of sorts. Physicians specializing in geriatrics say behavior patterns after the onset of Alzheimer's are influenced by each individual's disposition and temperment before the disease. But on one occasion Max insisted rather vigorously and vocally that "we get going, we have things to do."

Shortly after she said that, I had to take a business trip to Wichita. While there, I learned Max had come down with a terrible cold. Naturally, the threat of penumonia looms much larger for the elderly. I cut my trip short and flew back to Tucson the next day. Upon arriving, I drove straight to The Gardens. I saw Max walking up the hall and waved to her. She appeared to be well, but at our advanced ages, any kind of virus can be deadly serious business. Thank goodness professional caregivers are very aware of that.

The following afternoon I entered the home as Robin and Maxine were walking together, hand in hand. Max saw me and said, "You're not going to be mean to me, are you?" I said, "Of course not, my sweet. You are my precious -- I could never, ever be mean to you." She said, "That's good, because I love you so. . ."

As Max approached me, under the watchful eye and hand of Robin, I noticed some unsteadiness in her steps. In recent months she had been doing a lot of walking, yet I knew that it might be time for her to have the aid of a walker. I also knew, but hated to admit it, that eventually Max would require a wheelchair. I ordered a walker in mid-June 1999, and it was delivered within two weeks. At first it wasn't easy for Max to adjust, but once she got the hang of it, she shuffled all over the house.

While her movements were slow, Maxine became fairly adept at negotiating the long hallways with her new walker. She abruptly halted in the middle of her stride one day and almost collided head-on with a a pair of huge Dobermans held on leashes by another resident's daughter. Max didn't dislike dogs, she simply preferred they occupy someone else's space. She skirted around the animals and said, "They're nice, but now get them out of here!"

Max once owned a spotted cocker spaniel named Freckles -- just for the children, she maintained. Freckles had a roving eye and spent his days canvassing the neighborhood for unattached females. I'm sure he must have fathered more pups in Wichita than any other canine. However, before we married, I visited Maxine at her home, which, according to Freckles, was off-limits to all men but me. Any other male who came to the door was unceremoniously chased away amid loud barking, growling and ankle-snapping.

My brief visits to 111 Delrose seemed so distant after I took on the responsibility of a 24/7 caregiver in 1990. Today there's an organization called the National Family Caregivers Association (NFCA) whose objective is to bring greater recognition and rewards to family caregivers. I hadn't heard of NFCA, but had I known of its existence, it's doubtful I'd ever see it as my advocate.

I'm certain there's a place in our society for a consistant, well-coordinated effort supporting men and women engaged in heavily demanding home care of loved ones. Interestingly, the legions of unpaid caregivers are the ones who, unknowingly, pioneered the much-touted infrastrucure upon which our modern healthcare system has been developed. In my case, I sought absolutely nothing in return for my dedication to Maxine's daily care.

My commitment, of course, was to provide Maxine with her daily needs and do anything else that might improve her quality of life. One of NFCA's primary objectives was to ensure that home caregivers are given the same protection as the professionals, including the many thousands of certified aides in nursing homes. Whether federal or state, government regulations were intended to control and benefit the licensed employer of a nursing home.

According to NFCA, the state of affairs in home nursing is one of the most profound and widespread inequities attached to healthcare delivery in the United States. And initially, two of NFCA's principal targets were the Medicare and Medicaid programs. NFCA's goals are lofty, but in our nation's present political environment, it's unlikely reform can be achieved anytime soon.

For six of the eight years I served as Maxine's sole caregiver in our Green Valley home, I did all the cooking. It helped to know her likes and dislikes intimately, so I planned my menus accordingly. Shortly after moving to The Gardens, her eating habits became irregular, through no fault of the dieticians. Even so, Robin made sure Max received the proper nourishment with supplements and foods she enjoyed most, including large dishes of ice cream.

During the year I became acquainted with John Nighswander and his wife, Diana Will, both top executives at The Fountains, which owned and operated The Gardens and an assisted living apartment house called The Inn. One day we lunched together and I sensed all was not well in the ivory tower, and that the couple might opt for early retirement. I told Diana I'd always remember the day she saw Maxine's U of I certificate for the first time. She expressed her immediate reaction with one word: "Awesome!"

"Family Council" meetings, introduced by Robin, were held once a month in the evening. They were designed to exchange information between management and relatives of Alzheimer's residents. Mutual concerns were of primary importance. I attended religiously, but attendance was usually sparse. Some family members would distance themelves from the fact their loved ones had an incurable disease, missing opportunities for group discussions with their peers and residence director.

Rather than drive home in the dark after a council meeting, I'd stay overnight with Maxine. The first time I did that, as we prepared for bed, Max said, "Is it all right to do this, what will the others think?" I told her not to worry, we were married. She appeared much relieved.

CHAPTER 8

"I'm terrible - all mixed up."

Between visits with my beloved Maxine, I stayed busy, not so much un-bridled ambition as therapy for loneliness -- a diversion from sorrow, self-pity and the stark realization that Max was well beyond the point of no return (a flying term). Love is eternal, but the good Lord gave us only so many moments of togetherness. I missed more than ever the mutual comradeship we shared.

Ours had been a happy, mature, extremely deep relationship, a perfect anti-dote for the rigors of occupational pursuits. What I lacked now, most of all, was a true, intimate, trusty confidante. I had plenty of friends and relatives, yet no one could ever substitute for the distinctive character and exceptional qualities of my Maxine. She was irreplaceable.

More than once I thought of the only time our extended family saw Max simultaneously -- my three girls and her three, plus all the grandchildren, great grandchildren, nieces, nephew, a brother and sister-in-law. What had gotten us together (reunion style) was my enshrinement in the Arizona Aviation Hall of Fame (AAHF) in 1996. Joining us were many close friends and associates who came from far and wide to help celebrate the occasion.

I had reserved accommodations for 60 persons in the "Greenwood Group" at Embassy Suites near the Pima Air and Space Museum, site of the Arizona Aerospace Foundation's annual AAHF induction ceremony. Whenever a gang like this rallies around one of its own, there's bound to be a lot of kidding and ribbing about his or her deeds and misdeeds in years past.

Recapping one's journey through life clearly and concisely is challenging for even the most talented raconteur. My employment in the early days, I confess, was rather convoluted -- *Reader's Digest*, *The Washington Star*, *The Alexandria* (Virginia) *Gazette*, Goodyear Airship, United States Navy, Eastern Air Lines, *Miami Beach Florida Sun*, Miami All American Air Maneuvers, American Airmotive. All of these spanning the years 1938 to 1951.

Maxine and I often poked fun at each other, good naturedly, of course. After reviewing my checkered background in aviation one day early in our marriage, she turned to me and said, "For someone who couldn't hold a steady job, you haven't done too badly." She laughed at my retort: "Thanks, Sweetheart, I thought you were about to say that I was a classic example of how well our industry recycles its own waste."

I started out as a journalist, then merged two of my interests, flying and writing, when I went to work in aviation full-time. But newspapering was fun. For feature stories, I flew in a giant 10-engine B-36 nuclear bomber, inside the eye of a howling hurricane with the Navy, and through a complete air show in the back seat of an F-100F Super Sabre with the Air Force Thunderbirds jet aerobatic team. I rode in the slot position where you get a front row view of the leader's hot exhaust. Incidentally, I was the first person, civilian and military, to do this. And the last.

As a police reporter in Virginia and Florida, I encountered some interesting people, such as mob boss Meyer Lansky and his brother Jake. My counterpart on a rival Miami paper was the late Henry Reno, whose little daughter Janet grew up to become the U.S. attorney general. And Florida's top criminal defense lawyer, Benny Cohen, co-signed a bank note for me so I could buy an airplane, a war surplus Fairchild PT-19 primary trainer.

Life is filled with decision making -- and with people who in one way or another have had a tremendous impact on our lives. For example, as the fearless parachute jumper, I had performed in a few air shows with world aerobatic champion Bevo Howard. We became good friends and he later hired me as his assistant and coordinator of training at Hawthorne School of Aeronautics, a USAF primary flying school. Bevo had established the school to help the Air Force meet its pilot requirements for the Korean War.

In 1955, Beech Aircraft invited me to join its management team in Wichita, Kansas, widely heralded as an aircraft manufacturing center and the town Wyatt Earp reputedly tamed while serving as its constable. Bevo counseled me to accept the Beech offer since USAF contract pilot training's days were numbered. Had it not been for his advice, I might have gone off in some other direction and never met Maxine.

Nine years later, William Powell Lear, the aviation industry's "stormy genius," roared into Wichita like a tornado. He promptly raised some money with industrial bonds (the first ever in Kansas) and erected a factory for his new plane, the Learjet. He launched the company in Switzerland, then moved operations to Wichita where he could pirate the skills he needed from Beech, Boeing, and Cessna. I first met Bill in the forties, but resisted his overtures until early in 1964 when I finally capitulated and joined his jet set.

Again, had Bill Lear not been so persuasive in convincing me business travel's future lay in the small, pure jet, and not in the propjet as Beech predicted, I might have missed employing -- and marrying Maxine. I credit Lear's persistence in my seizing what he described as a "once-in-a-lifetime" opportunity.

At Learjet, Max had been more than an executive secretary. As a member of my corporate affairs staff, she played a dominant role in coordinating programs aimed at winning world acceptance of the small private jet. This included arranging international record attempts to help promote the safety, reliability, and utility of the light jet, as well as advances in turbojet technology. It was a fascinating, rewarding period in aviation history.

In 1970, three years after The Gates Rubber Company of Denver acquired Learjet, the Nixon administration asked me to accept an appointment to a high-level position in the FAA. Naturally, I was very proud to serve the president, but very glad when my stint with the Feds ended. I returned to Learjet in December 1973.

Though Max no longer worked for me as a company employee, she continued to be very helpful back in Wichita. I had a very capable staff at Learjet, but I relied on Maxine to edit all my paperwork for several major projects involving our airplane. First, I had charge of arranging the industry's first flying safety seminar for corporate jet owners and pilots. Second, as someone with solid FAA connections, I oversaw the company's successful effort to increase the Learjet's operating altitude from 43,000 to 51,000 feet, also an industry first.

My third important mission involved selecting a suitable site for plant expansion in the southwest. I picked Tucson in 1975, but never expected we'd ever relocate several corporate offices there, including mine. That happened in 1981 -- four years before I was scheduled to retire at the tender age of 65. Maxine was furious and in tears. She wanted no part of Arizona, which she imagined was Sahara Desert West. She even vented her feelings at Learjet's president, Harry Combs, a longtime friend and my boss.

Maxine and I had assisted Harry in writing his first book, the prize-winning *Kill Devil Hill: Discovering the Secret of the Wright Brothers*, with help from fellow writer Martin Caidin, who shared the byline. Combs acknowledged Max's contributions in the book, but went a bit further when he inscribed her personal copy: *"To my good friend Maxine Greenwood, whose insistence on accuracy made this book real. With grateful thanks, Harry Combs."*

In editing the manuscript, Max noted that Harry had slightly changed a number of the brothers' quotations to make them read "smoother, more euphonious." Max told Harry he couldn't do that, he had to quote the Wrights verbatim. She said someone would surely catch the alterations, and wrongly-worded quotes could impugn the integrity of the whole work. Harry fussed and fumed, but Max held her ground. After all was said and done, Combs gave in, not a single quote was changed. Harry respected Maxine's editorial judgment.

Now the shoe was on the other foot. Harry, mustering all of his abundant eloquence, set out to convince Maxine that once she was exposed to all the wonders and beauties of Arizona, she'd fall in love with the state. Max finally agreed to the move, but on one condition: we'd keep our house in Wichita and the day I retired we'd head for "home" with the speed of light. I concurred, and the wheels for our relocation were quickly set in motion.

We chose a small, compact house in an older section of Green Valley, an easy commute to our Tucson facility. Six months later, out of a clear blue sky, Maxine took me by the arm and said, "Don't you think it's time we sold our house in Wichita." Obviously, Max had become totally emersed in local community activities, including the AAUW, Illini Club and the Women's Club. And she was enjoying many new friends with common interests; our social calendar matched the one we had maintained in Wichita.

Meanwhile, we added 300 square feet to our Green Valley home's utility room, which Max labeled "The Last Re-sort." We needed the extra space mainly to accommodate my bulging files of aeronautical records, documents, speeches, news releases, awards, manuscripts, articles and pictures. When it came to collecting material, mostly paper, not even the prolific desert pack rat could touch us.

We had each vowed that the moment I retired, we'd both begin sorting out our overwhelming accumulation of "stuff," tossing all the printed matter not deemed absolutely essential. One day I saw Maxine diligently sifting through stacks of her papers, and every so often consigning something to one of several waste baskets. Not aware of me, she held up a single sheet of paper, studied it, then in all seriousness, said to herself aloud, "I guess I don't really need this, but I'd better make a copy of it first."

Jim Taylor, then Gates Learjet's president, told the anecdote at my Tucson retirement party in 1985. Good natured, gracious Max, who had realized her misstatement almost the instant she uttered it in my presence a few weeks earlier, laughed with the others as she heard it repeated for an audience. She saw humor in most things in life, even if the punchline bordered on self-depreciation. Yet she never made fun of others or joked at their expense.

That same year, the company generously honored us again with a second retirement bash held in New Orleans in conjunction with the National Business Aviation Association's annual convention. I was flattered by the turnout -- more than 500 friends and fellow workers in corporate aviation attended, many of them disbelieving that I was actually retiring. Charlie Gates, Harry Combs, Jim Taylor, and Neil Armstrong made the occasion especially memorable.

As a matter of fact, I didn't retire completely. The company retained me for two years as a consultant. Even after my contract expired, I continued working for myself as an aviation researcher, writer and technical advisor. Nobel Laureate James Watson, the co-discoverer of DNA structure, once said, "Never retire. Your brain needs exercise or it will atrophy."

Maxine accepted my thesis that we can extend the life of the body if we preserve the life of the mind. Exercising our intellect is vital to longevity. We're all living longer. Thanks to marked advances to science, medicine and genetic engineering, we can push well past the biblical limits of "threescore and ten." Unless, of course, we are struck down by some incurable disease that will kill us in the end.

In all the years since the doctors first diagnosed Maxine with Alzheimer's, caring for her had been my highest priority. Yet I felt it important, healthwise, to engage in several outside interests if and when possible. I had watched close friends slowly slip away, mostly because they did little or nothing constructive in the wake of their retirement.

My management services, aviation education and some historical preservation projects helped me maintain diversity and productivity in a drastically altered lifestyle. I also did ghostwriting for a few clients and accepted public speaking engagements, provided I knew something about the topic. While I found these activities to be mentally stimulating and personally satisfying, I never allowed them to interfere with my absolute dedication to Maxine's care.

I've also increased my understanding of Alzheimer's research and my support of efforts to find funding for it. Compared with other diseases, dementia studies have taken a backseat. Happily, the National Health Institute's spending for Alzheimer's research has been raised from around a half-billion dollars annually to more than a billion. Still, that's a drop in the bucket, considering the billions of dollars that go for AIDS, cancer, and arthritis.

Moreover, in keeping with its mission to conquer the disease, the Alzheimer's Association opposes any restriction or limitation on human stem cell research, but only if the appropriate scientific review, and ethical and oversight guidelines are in place. And I'm with Nancy Reagan who completely agrees with this new policy, which the AA's National Board of Directors adopted in 2004.

Cures for cancer, heart disease and stroke are on the way, and genetic engineering, stem cell regeneration, and organ transplants appear a certainty, all of which will have a favorable impact on life expectancy. Unfortunately, we're still searching for the best means of preventing or effectively treating Alzheimer's.

Researchers have made great strides in learning about causes and therapies, but much more work remains before we know enough to prevent Alzheimer's. Needed is the development of a broad spectrum of interventions for all stages of the disease. New drugs that can be used either alone or in combination with other recently approved medications may soon be available to halt the tide of what could become a worldwide Alzheimer's epidemic.

One of the newest drugs, memantine HCI (trade name Namenda™), seems to regulate the activity of glutamate, one of the brain's unique messenger chemicals. At normal concentrations, glutamate plays an essential part in learning and memory. Imbalances of gluatamate levels are believed to be one factor contributing to Alzheimer's-related memory problems and to the damage or destruction of nerve cells.

Memantine HCI's action in the glutamate system differs from the activity of four other cholinesterase inhibitors that are currently approved in the U.S. for treatment of Alzheimer's. Cholinesterase inhibitors temporarily boost levels of acetylcholine, another co-called messenger chemical that becomes deficient in the diseased brain of an Alzheimer's patient. Differing modes of action suggest that individuals might be able to take memantine HCI alone or with the other cholinesterase inhibitors.

In other research, experiments with mice offered hope that if a sticky brain plaque, amyloid beta peptide, is removed, the result might cure, or at least retard the disease. No one knows for sure if the plaque is the true cause of Alzheimer's, but it has become a prime suspect. Previously, scientists regarded plaque damage to nerve cells in the brain as something that happened once and was totally irreversible.

Researchers at Washingon University injected mice with an antibody vaccine that cleared plaque in parts of the brain. Where plaque was cleared, swelling on nerve cell branches disappeared quickly. Researchers cautioned, however, that while the treatment is most encouraging, more studies are required to learn if similar effects might occur in people.

Doctors tried dementia retardants on Maxine (as opposed to extreme or radical test procedures) in an unsuccessful attempt to slow the process of cognitive decline by breaking down the amyloid beta peptide buildup in the brain. But the medication had to be discontinued because one of the side effects aggravated her colitis problem. Also, her disease was considered much too far advanced for any meaningful testing.

University of Arizona and several other research centers in the U.S. are pioneering an approach to Alzheimer's that goes beyond treating symptoms. Their objective is outright prevention. They are working on a new track to iden-tify tests like brain scans or blood samples that could detect the disease long before symptoms even start. In fact, at this writing, a new treatment that would arrest a major cause of symptoms is undergoing clinical trials in Arizona and 15 other facilities in the U.S. and Canada. Scientists are so confident of its poten-tial they're calling it a vaccine.

MRI (magnetic resonance imaging) views of the brain's coronal sections reveal that Alzheimer's leads to severe degeneration in areas of the brain critical for memory, such as the hippocampus, a seahorse-like structure in the temporal lobes. Memory problems are the consequence of acute brain degeneration. A person suffering from Alzheimer's will have a greater amount of fluid-filled space around the entire brain -- and the fluid-filled ventricles are larger. How-ever, researchers disagree as to whether or not its the hippocampus or the frontal lobes that causes memories to resurface.

The medial temporal lobe, including the hippocampus, is the first place where damage appears in Alzheimer's victims. And that damage is responsible for the worst of the memory problems. Yet the frontal lobe is believed to be a major player in relating memories to personal experiences, which determines the details we remember in the first place. Some scientists believe it initiates the retrieval of old memories, acting as boss for the hippocampus. It's a fine theory, but is still subject to scientific debate.

Apart from the work being done on the brain, another, separate study con-firms that the loss of a loved one really can cause a broken heart. It found that grief or fear stimulates the adrenal glands and nerves, producing a surge of adrenaline and other stress hormones, resulting in a decline in the heart's pumping capacity. This reduction in pumping causes chest pain and other symptoms similar to heart attack.

I realized my own history of heart disease made me extremely vulnerable to anything that might affect my pump rate negatively. In some respects, I likened myself to someone standing on the edge of a precipice in a strong wind. And if I continued grieving, I could end up with "broken heart syndrome," technically known as stress cardiomyopathy. Consequently, I tried hard to keep my emotions, spirits, and mental outlook under control when I visited Maxine. Actually, her own cheerful disposition, despite the burden of Alzheimer's, made it easier for me.

For those of us still searching for answers, it was especially disheartening to learn that allegations of research misconduct had reached record highs in the closing years of the 20th century. One such case involved a renowned Alzheimer's researcher at the U of A in Tucson. Her widely publicized study showed that Vitamin E will delay aging of the immune system and the brain. But it proved to be without merit.

A regents professor in microbiology and immunology, the lady received worldwide attention for her "discovery," which resulted in a big run on Vitamin E supplements in the nation's drugstores. But alas, she lost her job after investigators found she had "falsified, manipulated, and otherwise misrepresented data and findings" in top medical journals and other publications.

Perhaps the most difficult thing for me to deal with was the pure and simple fact Max was aware that something was terribly wrong with her thought process, as well as her memory. We hardly ever discussed AD openly. She may not have known the root cause, but her perception of the problem came in loud and clear. "I'm terrible -- all mixed up," she said one morning. "There's something wrong with me, it's dreadful. I guess I'm almost out of it."

CHAPTER 9

"And who are you?"

Memories are priceless treasures. To have them stolen is one of Mother Nature's most heinous crimes against humanity. Memories nurture a positive outlook for those of us who might otherwise succumb to deep despair. In her best-selling book, *Pride and Prejudice*, author Jane Austen advises us to "Think only of the past as its remembrance gives you great pleasure." But Mark Twain put it another way: "Life would be infinitely happier if we could only be born at the age of eighty and gradually approach eighteen."

Indeed, Maxine was "all mixed up," in her words. Yet we've always held sacred our wedding vows: "... to have and to hold from this day forward, for better, for worse, for richer, for poorer, in sickness and in health, to love and to cherish, till death do us part."

Perhaps English author and poet Joseph Addison (1672-1719) put marriage more effusively when he wrote, "Two persons who have chosen each other out of all the species, with the design to be each other's mutual comfort and entertainment, have, in that action, bound themselves to be good humoured, affable, discreet, forgiving, patient, and joyful, with respect to each other's frailties and perfections, to the end of their lives."

I never held a single reservation about the daunting task of caring for my precious, even though in my case "closure and healing" were both illusions. The loss of a loved one to AD could not help but disrupt our lives, often making it difficult to handle other everyday problems. Reflecting on my own commitment, I knew in my heart of hearts that if the situation were reversed, Max would have been there for me in an instant. For ours was a loving, trust-filled, lifelong bond. And nothing nor anyone could ever change its dynamics.

Considering the circumstances, the hours I spent with Maxine at The Gardens were mutually rewarding. She laughed, or at least smiled, at my jokes and anecdotes. As we moved through autumn of 1999, I observed only a slight degradation in her overall condition and demeaner. While encouraging, I didn't let it raise any false hopes. The inevitable course for both of us had already been well charted by forces beyond our control.

There were days when caregivers described Maxine as "restless but cheerful." One day she greeted me by saying, "I'm glad you're here, otherwise I'd be zonked." Then she added, "I don't know who I am, where I am, or what I'm doing." Another time I talked about our "tieing the knot" in 1970, punctuating my brief soliloquy by saying, "Now you're stuck with me." She came right back with, "It's not 'stuck,' it's called love."

Then there were days when she was more confused, visibly tired and practically speechless. Her eating habits continued to waiver, as did her weight. She never refused ice cream, however. I saw to it that she received generous helpings of the frozen confection as frequently as possible. Visitations by family and friends were infrequent now, but always welcomed, especially if they came one at a time or in pairs. Occasionally I'd arrange for them to join us for a meal, when convenient to their schedules.

Maxine was always well groomed and manicured. At The Gardens we tried to maintain her pleasing appearance. The staff had a good selection of blouses, pants, sweaters, bras, panties, coats and jackets to choose from. (Though not totally incontinent, she wore protective undergarments just in case.) The caregivers saw to it that Max was always dressed comfortably and attractively. About them, she'd say, "Those girls are really good." And that may have been just 10 minutes after she had said, "Those girls are awful."

Max kept her pretty platinum blonde hair short and stylish, my favorite hairdo. Hilda Pesqueira, the beauty shop operator on the premises, trimmed it every four weeks. I made sure her nails, chin whiskers, hair and clothes were always presentable. A local podiatrist, Dr. Larry Wessel, stopped in every two months and cut Maxine's toenails.

Some years before AD we visited Marquita and Loren Brown and I sported a fresh crewcut, somewhat shorter than usual. One summer afternoon the sun struck it just right as we were getting in the car with our three-year-old grandson Taylor Brown. Taylor looked at my very short hair and said, "Grandpa, your hair's all gone." Maxine, whose hair was snow-white, asked Taylor, "What about my hair, grandma's hair?" The child responded, "You've got old hair." Maxine thought that was funny and often repeated it.

During one of her regular visits, Dr. Tenney Kentro's nurse, Andy Colussi, said Max appeared more disoriented than usual that day and ordered more blood work. A few days later the lab report came in with good news: All tests were negative. Also that day, I got out Maxine's memory book and showed her where we honeymooned at the Fredericksburg Inn in Fredericksburg, Virginia. I said, "Our friend Syd Shannon, the owner, gave us the bridal suite." Max studied the picture, then said, "And when was I 'bridled'?"

It happened to be September 11, 1999, our 29th anniversary, so I turned to our wedding pictures. Since we both had colds, I told Max we'd celebrate quietly. "Oh," she said, "and just who are we?" I couldn't suppress a laugh, so I flipped the pages until I came to the photos of our Acapulco fishing trip, which she had already seen many times. Soon as Max saw her picture kneeling beside the 187-pound sailfish she boated, she touched it and said, "This is a riot -- is it true?"

My daily routine had fallen into a pattern. My visits with Max alternated between mornings and afternoons. Frequently I would stay for lunch (actually dinner, the main meal) or supper, which usually consisted of fruit, sandwich, drink and dessert. By dining with Max, I relieved whichever caregiver had been assigned to feed her, if she balked at eating that particular day.

I always checked the activities calendar in advance, even though Maxine became increasingly disinterested in participating in the scheduled events. She seemed more at ease with me alone in her room where I had access to an ample supply of reading material. Maxine herself had lost the ability to read more than a few words at a time, and even then her attention span was receding. In fact, she had no interest in television. But she still enjoyed leafing through the pages of magazines, often tearing out some of them. Robin would say, "It looks like Maxine is editing again."

Maxine's chest X-rays, taken earlier, were negative. Robin and I were afraid she might have developed a lung infection. Some strong antibiotics and decongestants that had been prescribed for her did the trick. As everyone at The Gardens knew, I was always concerned about her medication and I monitored it closely.

Maxine didn't feel well December 14 and wanted to stay in bed. She coughed repeatedly at breakfast, yet managed to eat most of the meal. When I arrived, I found Max sitting in the foyer, one of her favorite places at The Gardens. She quizzed me about who I was and whether I really belonged to her. Robin stopped by and gave me a copy of the lab report on Maxine's most recent blood tests, which were negative.

Fifteen minutes later Dr. Kentro visited us and tried hard to examine Maxine while she rested in her room. He didn't have much success, as Max was too fidgety. He said her glucose count was out of range, probably because her blood specimen was taken right after a breakfast of pancakes and syrup, which she devoured. And more sonic tests and X-rays of Maxine's abdominal area were ordered by the doctor. As I was leaving, Max asked me if we could go home. I said, "We are home." Max: "That's good."

I had told Max about the new millennium, now a little over two weeks away. I said the dictionary defines a millennium as a period of "righteousness and happiness," especially as it pertains to the "indefinite future." She wasn't the least bit impressed. Anyway, the mainstream press was making it a big deal, referring to it as Y2K, which became its popular designation.

Since there was a lot of speculation as to what surprising and terrifying consequences we might expect at midnight 1999, I thought I'd better record the event for the family, if not posterity. As the reader must know by now, I kept copious notes to document Max's care and physical and mental condition. The following entries from by daily journals cover the last week of 1999, leading up to the turn of the century. The text has been edited for brevity, but all the quotations herein are verbatim, just as they are everywhere else in this book:

December 24 -- Christmas Eve party a big success. (My daughter, Roxanne Cable, with us for the holidays.) We arrived in the afternoon: Max met me and asked, "Are you yourself?" I said yes. Maxine: "I'm so happy you're here." Everyone, staff and residents alike, was in the Yuletide spirit. Management had gifts for residents and relatives. We (Roxie, Maxine and I) sat with Susan and her mother, Ethel Jacobs, a resident. Max ate her share of "goodies," but was impatient to "get going." I said we'd leave for home as soon as Roxie finished eating. Max turned to Roxie and said, "Can you hurry, please!" Several caregivers sang "Jingle Bells" and a few of us joined in, whether on or off key. Back in the room, I read Maxine's personalized booklets. She laughed at the passages mentioning her name.

"And who are you?"

December 25 -- Christmas. Sharon said Maxine up most of the night, only had about an hour's sleep. Jaime Henson, Robin's daughter, said girls working split shifts today, enabling everyone to enjoy at least part of Christmas with their families. Roxie and I had Christmas dinner with Maxine, then opened our presents. (Max, with help from Robin, made me a small bouquet of paper flowers in a little flower pot.) At one point today, Max looked at me and said, "I won't let you out of my sight." She also complained about tummy cramps, after consuming almost everything on her plate. We went to Max's room and I gave her a purple pill. Roxie took a walking tour of The Fountains' campus while Max and I rested. I sang songs, told jokes and got her laughing again.

December 26 -- Pat said Maxine given a suppository this morning and has since had a small BM. She's improved today. Drove Roxie to the airport for return flight to Austin. I went back to The Gardens where Max had been resting, but I got her up for pie and ice cream in the dining room. She asked about children, then remarked, "Come and live with our family." I walked into another room looking for Maria and heard my Maxine calling out, "You who, you who!" Max did not want me to go to the office and repeatedly said, "Stay with me!" I told her Virginia and Maria (caregivers) would keep her company until I got back. But my reasoning didn't work as well today as it had in the past.

December 27 -- Jaime said Robin and Carla had to help get Maxine up this morning, though the night shift did not report anything indicating a bad night. She ate a good breakfast of eggs, sausage, juice and toast, and about three-fourths luncheon pizza. (Jaime's developed a warm personal relationship with Max, which is good.) Jaime saw to it that Max drank all of her supplement, a chilled can of strawberry Equate, which she loves.

Decmeber 28 -- Max ate all her breakfast then asked Pat, "Where's my father?" Pat said, "You mean Jim?" Max: "Yes." Pat told her I'd be there soon and she grinned. As I arrived,

Max saw me getting out of the car and told Heather, "That looks like my father." Heather brought her outside to meet me. She waved as I approached her. Inside we stopped at Robin's office for a briefing on Thursday's visit to Northwest for lab tests (sonogram). While talking to Robin, Max suddenly said, "I'm going to kiss you." And she did. Showed Max latest Xmas cards and the book we co-authored (SFITM). Gertrude came to Max and MiMi's room and somehow slipped to the floor. I didn't try to pick her up. Maria and Jaime were able to get her up. No hurts, but Jaime herself has all the symptoms of a bad cold or the flu.

December 29 -- Yolanda reported Maxine up late again. She's in good spirits today. Max, standing in dining room with another resident, spotted me and asked, "Are you my father?" I said, "I'm your husband, Jim" She said, "Of course. I want to go with you now." Nicole Getker came with me to see Max. The three of us went to the office and chattted briefly with Robin, Kathleen, Maria, Kimberly. Max grew impatient. She said loud and clear, "Let get going!"

December 30 -- Arrived at 8:30 a.m. Kathleen had Max ready for drive to Northwest for additional sonogram testing. Robin was a great help; she accompanied us. (Don't think I could have done it without her.) Back at the residence, Kathleen changed Maxine's clothes, which had become soiled from the cream used for sonic tests. (Results were negative.) I left at noon.

December 31 -- Heather told Max I'd be there in the afternoon and planned to remain overnight. On duty today: Robin, Margarita, Virginia, Jaime, Kimberly. (Heather at B, but still punky.) Today historically significant. It marks the end of the 20th century. Tomorrow, January 1, 2000, is the start of the new 21st century, referred to as Y2K (the new millennium actually begins in 2001). Max and I dined together (she ate 100 percent), then enjoyed a "New Year's Eve party" arranged by Margarita and Virginia. Good music, snacks. Margarita and I each made some semblance of "dancing" with Max, who wasn't at all interested in moving her feet in step with the music. As we got ready for bed (with Virginia's help), I once again told Max about the U of I classroom to be named in her honor. I said, "Nothing has ever been named for me." Max quickly replied, "Yes it has -- me!"

We were in bed by 9 p.m. for a memorable night. Told Max to sleep tight and not let the bedbugs bite. She said, "They'd better not." Next I recited an age-old bedtime prayer: "Now I lay be down to sleep, I pray the Lord my soul to keep. If I should die before I wake, I pray the Lord my soul to take." Max followed me through it the second time and did quite well. As we settled down in her bed, she snuggled up and even put her arm around me, just like she used to. All of a sudden she asked, "And who are you?"

Max was only up twice during the night. (I was up no less than four times.) Sharon Warren came in at 6:30 to get Max up, washed and dressed. Max and I were at the breakfast table by 8. Carla and Kathleen were the caregivers on duty. Max ate pancakes and sausage, an extra pancake, glass of milk, and three glasses of fresh orange juice. I pottied Max, then we sat in the foyer. For me, this visit was especially touching, but I had to go. Max said, "I'll go with you, because I don't want you to leave me." I told her Carla and Kathleen would keep her company while I was at the office, but I'd be back."

Despite widespread concerns that the calendar change -- 1999-2000 -- would cause some sort of cybernetic catastrophy, the global transition at midnight went smoothly and quietly in all time zones. The whole notion that computers everywhere would crash, whether they were turned on or not, was the product of fanatics who fed an overly gullible news media with misinformation on the state of the electronic sciences. We were told bank records would be wiped out, businesses would collapse, and all machinery powered by electric generators would come to a complete standstill.

Particularly scary was a warning that the international air traffic control system would shut down, causing thousands of planes to lose their way and run into each other. Younger caregivers, who grew up in the age of cyberspace, were especially vulnerable. They became extremely alarmed by what they had read and heard. I tried to calm them, and believe I succeeded to some extent.

On the morning of New Year's Day, I told the staff "millenary mania" was over. The earth was still spinning at 1,000 miles an hour and no one had fallen off, nor had even a drop of ocean been spilled. I said 1,000 years ago Y1K came and went with no adverse effects. So did Y2K, in spite of all the hysteria surrounding it. Then I added, "The 21st century is here, ready or not."

Because of Alzheimer's, Maxine was spared millennium madness. She also was spared far worse events that came later, including earthquakes, tsunamis and other natural disasters. She missed the war on terrorism and other examples of man's inhumanity to man at home and abroad. And she was totally unaware of al-Qaida's attacks on New York and Washington on September 11, 2001 -- our 31st wedding anniversary. Five days later a pilot was killed when he crashed his Cessna into a house three blocks from Maxine's.

During the first few years of the 21st century, the repetition of disturbing news was almost too much: Societal moral decay, more assaults on our core beliefs, political and fiscal corruption at the highest levels, drug trafficking, and illegal immigration, plus an increasing toll on human life due to conflicting cultures, ideas, and causes that were running rampant everywhere. Our world seemed clearly divided into two camps -- good and evil, each with its own legions of idealists and functionaries.

Care home residents exposed to all this doom and gloom in the mainstream media became emotionally distraught and unstable, though their agitation lasted only as long as they had access to newspaper headlines, radio and television. Maxine, of course, was somewhat insulated. I realized I could never create a feeling of euphoria in place of fear, but I was determined to shield her troubled mind from anything unpleasant or provocative for as long as she lived.

CHAPTER 10

"She has a nice smile."

For me, the year 2000 was a bittersweet mixture of emotional highs and lows. On the upside, the dedication of "Maxine's Classroom" on May 9 at the University of Illinois was inarguably the year's most memorable event. The worst downer was an increasing concern over management problems at The Gardens. Also, Max's health appeared to be losing ground slowly but steadily. Early in the year her weight had dropped to 100 pounds, the lowest since she was first diagnosed with Alzheimer's. And another sonic test of her abdomen disclosed a collapsed gall bladder.

Certain staff conflicts, personal animosities and a general misunderstanding of key corporate policies at The Gardens resulted in disciplinary actions and, in some extreme cases, dismissals. Moreover, Robin's support from top management kept eroding. The Gardens, an Arizona state model for memory care when it opened in January, 1998, appeared to be slipping off its pedestal.

Robin saw the situation as untenable, and, regrettably, turned in her resignation, effective June 30. She had been in demand for sometime within the healthcare management community and elected to accept what she considered to be the most attractive offer. With Robin's departure, The Fountains, assisted living facility, called The Inn, and the two AD units, Casa Allegra and Casa Bonita -- paired together as The Gardens -- lost a valuable asset, one management found extremely hard to replace.

On a more positive note, I had the pleasure of dedicating The H. Maxine Gladding Greenwood Video Editing Suite in the College of Communications,

University of Illinois at Urbana-Champaign. Max, of course, couldn't attend because of her disease. But, as I told those present for the ceremonies, she was with us in spirit, looking over our shoulders to make sure we did everything right.

An ancillary benefit was the opportunity to meet, for the first time, members of Max's extended family. Dean Kim Rotzoll of the College of Communications had invited her relatives, most of whom still lived in the area. I knew Max's brothers, Don and George Gladding, but the cousins and other kin I'd never met before. They were prone to treat me like the family's long-lost favorite uncle. And their enthusiasm for my project was most gratifying.

Bernie Freeman's talent for organization surfaced again when she arranged an intensive, hour-by-hour itinerary for my four-day visit. Suffice to say, I saw more of the University's magnificent campus in four days than the average student sees in four years. Everywhere I went, the warm hospitality and many other courtesies extended me by U of I staff and faculty reinforced my original decision to honor my beloved wife in some tangible way at her alma mater, where she had distinguished herself academically.

Dean Rotzoll chaired a brief program held in a Gregory Hall conference room, followed by a tour of the classroom site in the same building. Mitch Kazel of the Journalism faculty conducted the tour, explaining all the complexities of video editing in today's age of instant communications.

Needless to say, I was fascinated by Kazel's description of the suite's electronic sophistication. When I practiced journalism in the days before and immediately after World War II, print media was my forté. Broadcast news sources were limited to radio at that time, though television had already been invented and soon dominated the air waves. Next, cybernetics emerged, giving the world a wide range of communications options.

Television news and other TV programming will be with us far into the future. And it takes dozens of qualified technicians to back up TV news producers, on-camera commentators, and anchors. But none has a more important role than the video editor. He or she must forge the daily material into a specific format within the news show's time frame. Editing video news is a highly skilled and demanding profession, one requiring extensive training.

Mitch Kazel told our group Maxine's new suite contains four individual sound-proofed, temperature-controlled studios used by broadcast journalism students and faculty for traditional tape-based and non-linear digital video editing. A fifth "equipment room" features satellite downlink facilities for CNN

Newsource and remote program origination equipment for UI-7, the cable TV service of the University of Illinois. A lobby area has work space for a student lab monitor, three battery-charging stations, and storage cabinets for video camcorders, tripods and other accessories.

"This suite consolidates student video editing in one location, replacing a small inadequately partitioned and non-air-conditioned classroom that served as a makeshift editing lab for almost twenty years," said Kazel. "This is a modern, comfortable facility that will serve the needs of our students every day of class for many years to come."

As I said at a special luncheon in the Student Union, the new facility and what it means to the University is a dream come true. To say I was impressed by its broad capabilities would be a gross understatement. I had no idea students planned to use the classroom 24 hours around the clock when nearing deadlines. Just imagine going to class at 2 or 3 in the morning.

During lunch, Maxine received one accolade after another in absentia. Dean Rotzoll also mentioned our deferred gift for the H. Maxine Gladding Greenwood Award, and recognized Don Gladding's contribution of $25,000 toward the cost of upgrading all the equipment in his sister's new suite. I responded by saying Maxine would probably disapprove of all the fuss being made over her. On the other hand, she'd be very proud too -- and humbled -- by the eulogies.

The Green Valley News and Sun, our local newspaper, published a long illustrated article about Maxine shortly after I returned home. Headlined Legacy of Love, the feature story recognized Max's remarkable achievements under extremely difficult circumstances. As usual, I had stayed in touch with Casa Allegra by phone while I was away, but couldn't wait to see Max upon my return.

My unbridled exhilaration over the week's activities in Urbana was tempered by the realization Maxine might not fully understand the underlying significance of what we had done for the University. Anyway, my homecoming was heartening. Soon as Maxine saw me, she extended her arms and clapped.

I read a story about her in one of the U of I's publications and she said, "That's lovely." Then I showed Max a photo of me unveiling her bronze plaque at the dedication ceremony. It hangs on the wall at the entrance to her classroom. Titled the H. Maxine Gladding Greenwood Video Editing Suite, it features her portrait and a brief inscription which reads:

"Inspired by her commitment, hard work and determination,
James R. Greenwood proudly dedicates this suite to honor his

beloved wife Maxine, University of Illinois Journalism Class
of 1938 and a Bronze Tablet Scholar."

A few weeks later, I was prepared to show Max all the pictures and articles
about her. Besides the local newspaper, university publications that featured
Maxine and our philanthropy included *Investing in Illinois*, *The College of
Communications Alumni News*, and the *University of Illinois Foundation
Generations*.

Each of the pieces provided extensive coverage, editorially and pictorially.
I arrranged all the material in a special U of I album as a companion to Maxine's
memory book, including the most prolific letters of commendation Max received
from friends, family and even a few strangers. Showing her my favorite photo,
Maxine said, "Is that me, really?" I said, "Yes, you're still my pretty sweetheart." Flipping over to another picture, I said, "That's you too." Max studied it,
then said, "She has a nice smile."

On October 3, 2002, the U of I's College of Communications celebrated
"75 years of excellence" as a separate school, although journalism instruction
there actually began in 1902. The college's timeline brochure, denoting important milestones in its history, carried this entry for May 9, 2002:

> "The H. Maxine Gladding Greenwood Video Editing Suite in
> the basement of Gregory Hall is dedicated. Maxine, who gradu-
> ated in 1938, can't attend because of Alzheimer's, but her husband,
> Jim, is there to see how their $100,000 gift transformed the
> former classroom space into a modern editing suite for broad-
> cast students, thanks to the efforts of Mitch Kazel, teaching
> associate."

Bernie Freeman and Jeff Roley of the University of Illinois Foundation,
and Dean Kim Rotzoll, visited Maxine whenever possible while in the Tucson
area. Rotzoll, in fact, made two special trips to The Gardens, one of them with
his wife Nancy shortly before the classroom dedication. For that special occasion, we dressed Max in her new T-shirt reading, "College of Communications,
University of Illinois," which Kim had sent to her earlier. Max was all smiles
and held Nancy's hand as a token of her esteem.

Working with Dean Rotzoll on the classroom project was a sheer delight.
His support, guidance, and insistance on quality throughout the whole process

was inspiring and reassuring. We remained in close contact during the construction phase. And Kim's progress reports kept me well informed of every last detail, from classroom concept right on down to its furnishings. By the time it was all over, I felt like a U of I alumnus emeritus.

As my friends at the U of I know, Maxine's disease robbed her of long-term, as well as short-term, memory. Yet mentioning Maxine's undergraduate days at the University of Illinois always triggered a fleeting expression of recognition. As the classroom was being built, Kim and I exchanged correspondence and telephone calls. His notes to us, short and sweet, were gems. One was very special and touched us both. It simply said, *"Jim, you and your beloved are a class act."*

Kim Rotzoll's untimely death on November 4, 2003, left a giant void at the University. However, the powers-that-be wisely chose Ron Yates, a veteran newspaperman and head of the Department of Journalism, as Rotzoll's successor. Replying to my letter of congratulations, Dean Yates wrote: "Obviously, having state-of-the-art facilities such as the H. Maxine Gladding Greenwood Video Editing Suite is critical to us. It is a wonderful facility, and I can assure you it is populated with students almost every hour of every day during the school year."

Back in the world of dementia after a most enjoyable respite in academe, I reflected on how and why all this got started. It was actually over breakfast with a dear friend and colleague during one of my infrequent trips to Wichita. Al Higdon, my associate at Beech and Learjet, was well aware of my interest in providing a living tribute that would honor my beloved Maxine in an appropriate and enduring manner.

We discussed the increasing importance of private donations in helping colleges and universities establish and maintain leadership roles in higher education. Private donations provide the resources to fund new construction, equip laboratories, endow chairs, support students, underwrite research, and enrich the educational experience of students in innumerable ways.

Following my conversation with Al, I contacted the University of Illinois Foundation and within a couple of weeks I was meeting with Bernie Freeman and Jeff Roley in the offices of my attorney, Tim Olcott. They said a deferred grant to fund scholarships would be most welcomed, but asked me to consider the most urgent need in the College of Communications' Department of Journalism -- a new video editing suite.

I liked the immediacy of honoring Maxine now, while she was still living, so I decided to do both. Consequently, a greater number of students seeking careers in video editing will benefit directly and immediately from an outright gift toward a new suite. No longer would enrollment be limited because of inadequate classroom space and equipment. Naturally the U of I is also most grateful for the endowment we established. And eventually, upon my demise, it will fund student scholarships and faculty awards.

Why did I do this? Maxine had been such a vibrant, vital part of my life I wanted to honor her in some special, personal way. When you adore someone as much as I loved, admired, and respected Maxine, the most sincere, romantic motivation springs straight from the soul. The rest is history.

Shortly after the Legacy of Love feature appeared in our local newspaper, we received many complimentary letters, each saying what a wonderful thing we had done. Bill Robinson wrote, "This will be a living memorial in Maxine's name that will be remembered for many years." Al and Judy Higdon's brief note capsulized Maxine's warmth and character clearly and incisively:

> *To Our Dear Friend Maxine,*
>
> *We remember when we first met, so many years ago, because of a marvelous company filled with wonderful people;*
>
> *We remember your kindness in paying a call to our home to help welcome our first-born child into the world;*
>
> *We remember many special visits to places near and far away, renewing old times and making new ones;*
>
> *Most of all we remember your smile, your helpful words and your enthusiasm for life.*
>
> *Maxine, you are truly one of God's best. Our lives are enriched by being able to call you our friend.*
>
> *Judy and Al Higdon*

I read and re-read the Higdon letter to Maxine, who showed no visible emotion at first. Then I reminded her that Al and I had shared many exciting experiences working together. And she, Maxine, helped us. I said our big job was to convince companies with far-flung travel requirements that they needed the flexibility and high performance of a private jet -- the Learjet. Suddenly Max interrupted me and said, "Yes, I know him, is he here?"

Overall, June 2000 was a rather eventful month. One afternoon gave me quite a scare. I arrived at The Gardens just after Robin had finished rinsing out Maxine's mouth. It seems that one of the new caregivers got distracted while removing the polish from Max's nails. Max promptly picked up the bottle of polish remover and put it to her lips. Robin saw this and quickly intervened. It's not likely that Maxine swallowed any of the liquid, thanks to Robin's lightning-fast action.

However, the incident was another alarming reminder to the staff that caregivers using any kind of potentially injurious substance in the vicinity of persons with AD must never let their attention be diverted, even for an instant. Polish remover contains ethyl acetate and other harmful ingredients. If taken internally, according to the doctors, it can cause nausea and vomiting.

On a happier note, my three daughters, Roxanne, Jeanne and Karen, surprised me with a special five-day holiday at the famous Colony Beach and Tennis Resort on Florida's Longboat Key in honor of my 80th birthday. It was a welcomed, relaxed diversion and it gave me a chance to sort out the large bodies of information in my mind and organize them in such a way as to give me a clearer picture of the problems and a working hypothesis for their solution.

While there, we drove our rental car over to nearby Sarasota Bradenton International Airport, so I could show the girls where I made my last exhibition parachute jump in 1949. It was a small field back then, but interestingly, the airport's original flying service, Jones Aviation, was still there, though much bigger and more expansive in its operations. And I renewed my acquaintance with its president, Clyde Jones, who remembered all the details of our airshow 51 years before, including a delinquent fuel bill. (*Author's note:* The three girls came to Arizona for my 85th in 2005, but the venue lacked many of the features of Longboat Key. They were contemplating something similar for my 90th. However, I suggested they think in terms of an annual birthday observance from now on. At my age, I'm a target for too many crippling attacks on my health.)

During the month, Vivienne also blessed us with a surprise visit, toting Mother's Day and Father's Day presents, which we opened after a tasty lunch. She had not seen managing editor Kathy Engle's Legacy of Love article in the *Green Valley News and Sun*, so she proceeded to read it aloud for her mother, whose facial expression revealed curiosity. With her eyes fixed on the paper, Max pointed to her picture and said, "She looks cheerful."

Vivie came to the end of the story, and Maxine said, "You know something,

I don't believe it." Vivie and I both told Max it was all true. Max said, "It is, well okay, that's good." Just before Vivie left, Max got on her bed with a little help and called out to me, "Jim, Jim, I'm ready for you now," meaning she wanted me to lay down beside her. I did, then I got up to hug and kiss Vivienne goodbye, as she was leaving. It was the first time I had ever seen Max show any sign of jealousy over anyone, much less her own daughter. Max exclaimed, "Jim, come here. I don't like you doing that!"

Shortly before her departure, Robin informed the Casas Allegro and Bonita family councils of her new position -- director of Alterra Healthcare's Sterling House, an assisted living residence several miles north of The Gardens. Robin understood my growing concerns and primarily wanted to stress that steps were being taken to remedy any problems I had voiced.

Until a suitable replacement for Robin was hired, caregivers at houses A and B in The Gardens would report to supervisors at The Inn or The Fountains, not exactly a desirable chain of command when dealing with dementia victims. Robin also recommended Maxine stay put until I saw how her successor performed. Unfortunately, there would be several successors, including the overseeing supervisors already designated, serving as "directors" before I might face another tough decision involving a residence change, if it came to that.

Meanwhile, Maxine's eating habits had improved slightly, along with her weight. So far, management's budget cutting had not yet impacted the quality or quantity of the meals. Inevitably it might and indeed it did. I had already discussed the situation at The Gardens with Michael Hughes and Mary Joe Erickson of the Fountains executive staff, both of whom assured me that all the concerns of family members were being addressed.

However, I went back to Diana Will and John Nighswander, who had just retired from top postions at The Fountains, though both were still available to the company as consultants. John was very candid about his "retirement." He had served the corporation almost from the beginning and contributed much to its growth. His wife Diana, likewise, had been a valued, longtime employee.

John heard me out, then responded by saying he had seen a widening breach in management philosophy, a new direction he found unacceptable. Over his objections, the company instituted certain cost-reduction measures that inpinged on the high standard of services rendered at both The Inn and The Gardens. Apparently, John's counter recommendations for achieving operational economies in other areas had fallen on deaf ears.

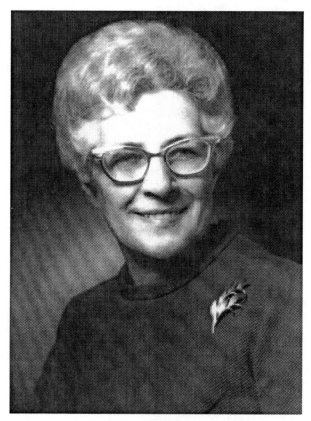

Maxine Greenwood

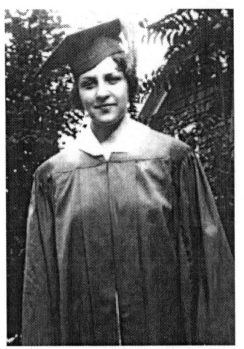

*Maxine ready for Urbana
High School graduation, 1934.*

*Portrait taken in 1937, one year
before graduating from
University of Illinois.*

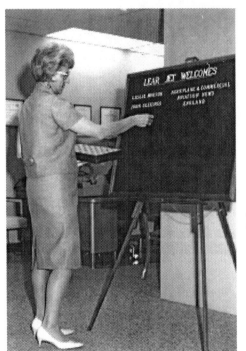

*Maxine posting names of
visiting journalists at Learjet,
1965.*

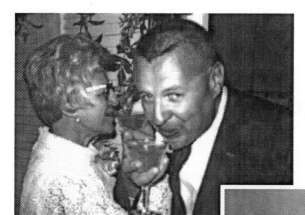

Traditional toast celebrating their marriage.

Vows sealed with a kiss at wedding reception.

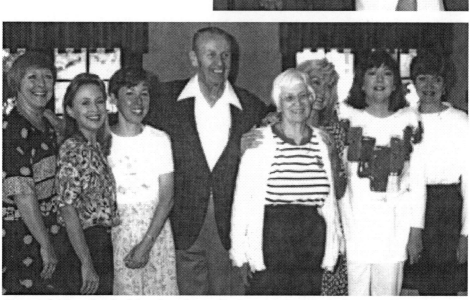

Jim and Max flanked by daughters. Left to right: Jim's Jeanne, Roxanne and Karen; Maxine's Yvonne, Marquita and Vivienne, 1996.

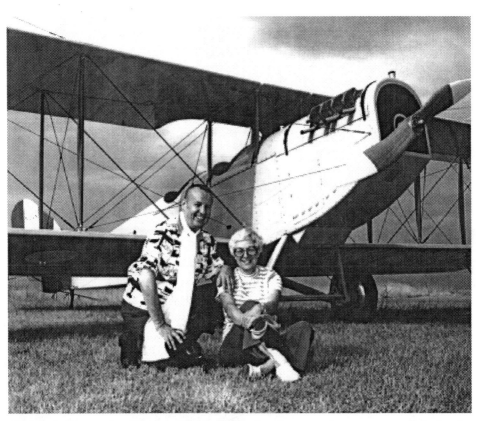

Sitting in front of a Curtiss JN-4D Jenny in photo used to promote their book,
Stunt Flying in the Movies.

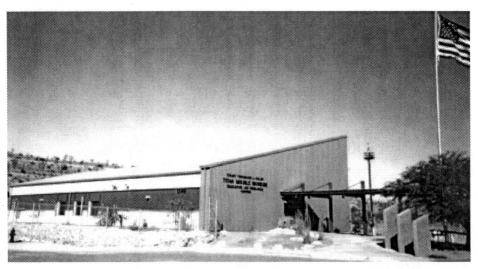

Titan Missile Museum at Sahuarita, Arizona, houses The Jim and Maxine
Greenwood Aerospace Education Center.
Its credo:"Not everyone can teach, but everyone can learn."

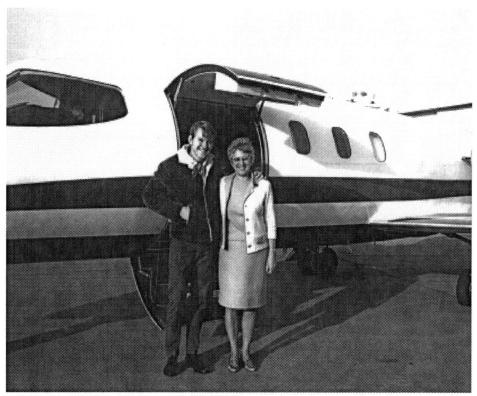

Maxine and Eric Blum of Twentieth Century-Fox, who represented the studio in special projects involving LearJet.

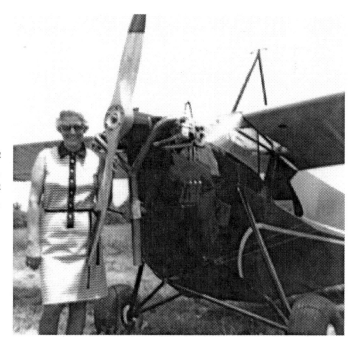

Max poses with Aeronca C-3, a type Jim flew in the late 1930s.

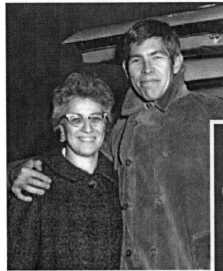

With actor James Coburn, during his Wichita factory visit.

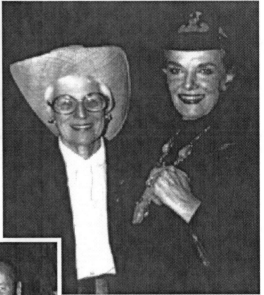

The Greenwoods were guests of actress Jane Russell in her California home.

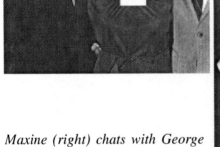

With Neil Armstrong at Jim's retirement party in New Orleans, 1985.

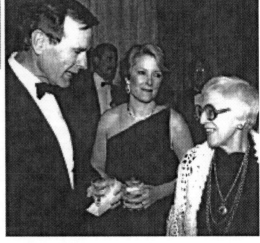

Maxine (right) chats with George Bush, then Vice President, at Wright Memorial ceremonies, honoring Harry Combs, 1985.

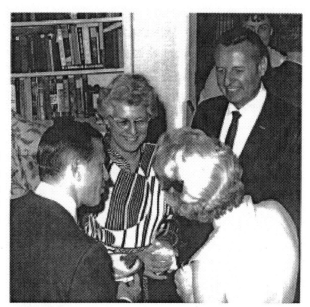

Max and Jim with Transportation Secretary John Volpe (left) at Jean Ross Howard's private reception.

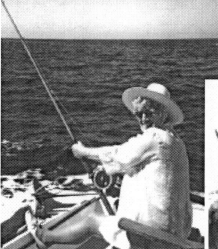

Max had never fished before, but agreed to hold a pole in Pacific waters off Acapulco.

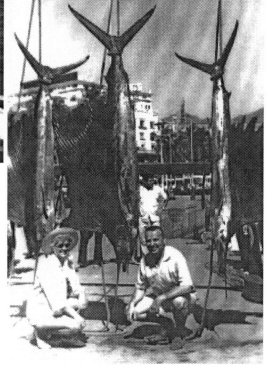

Result: She boated a 10-foot long, 187-pound sailfish (center), all by herself.

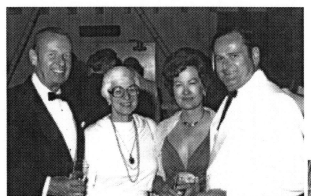

Jim, Max, Donna and Hoot Gibson, Korean jet ace and leader of the USAF Thunderbirds, when Jim flew with the jet team in 1962.

Aboard an old whaler moored firmly to the dock.

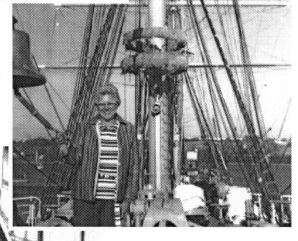

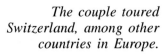

Maxine enjoyed traveling; here she is in England, 1972.

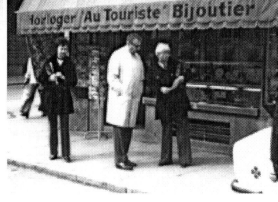

The couple toured Switzerland, among other countries in Europe.

Max tries a horse at an historic ranch in Arizona.

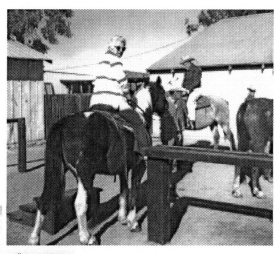

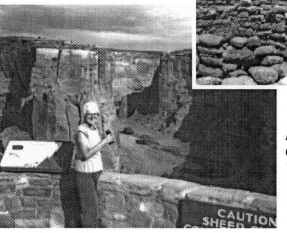

Finding an ancient Indian wall with Jim Pollock (left) and hubby Jim.

Exploring Indian ruins became a favorite pastime.

First visit to the Grand Canyon evoked one word, "Awesome."

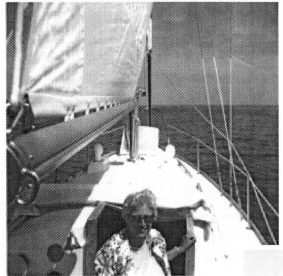

Aboard a new sloop in the middle of the Chesapeake Bay.

Jim and Max revisit the Old Presbyterian Meeting House 25 years after their 1970 wedding there.

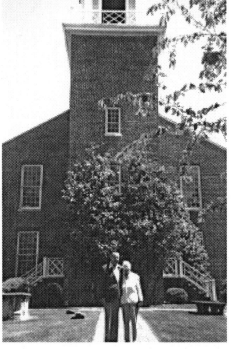

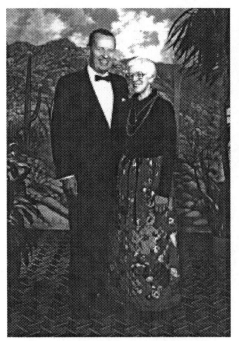

Max and Jim at the annual Angels Ball formal in Tucson, Arizona.

Front entrance to The Garden's Casa Allegra, Maxine's first "home away from home."

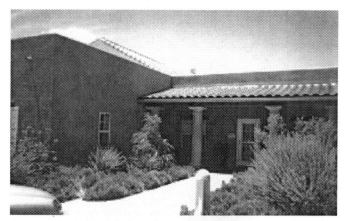

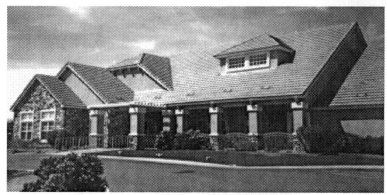

Resembling an English manor house, The Place at Tucson was Maxine's last home.

With daughter Marquita Brown and grandaughter Brittney, age 11.

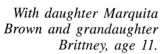

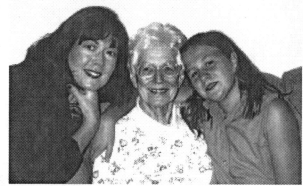

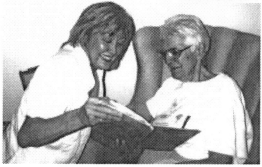

Eldest daughter Yvonne Duarte reads to her mother during a periodic visit.

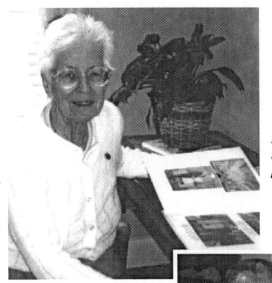

Maxine enjoyed her "memory book," opened here to wedding pictures.

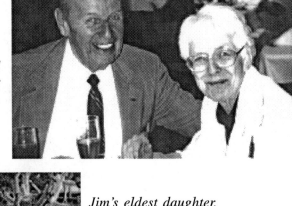

Jim and Max at a special dinner at The Inn, next door to The Gardens.

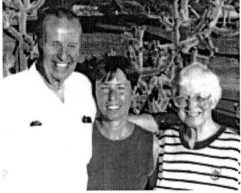

Jim's eldest daughter, Karen Kraus, during a 1996 trip to Green Valley.

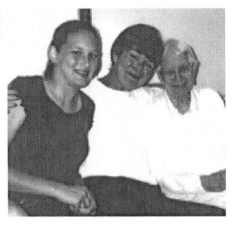

Granddaughter Michele and daughter Vivienne Sargeant with granny Maxine.

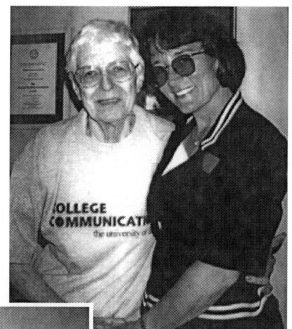

With director Robin Henson at The Gardens. Note gym shirt, a gift from the University of Illinois.

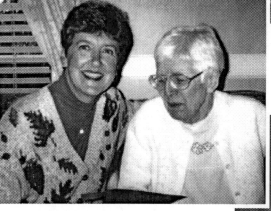

Bernie Freeman gives Maxine a U of I pennant, later posted next to door outside her apartment.

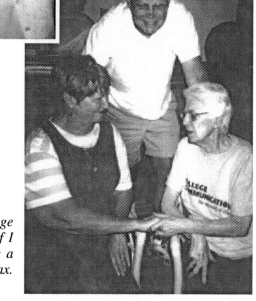

Dean Kim Rotzoll of College of Communications at U of I and wife Nancy made a special trip to see Max.

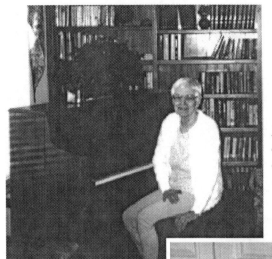

Maxine sat down at the piano on her own in The Place and actually tried to play.

Jim's daughter Roxanne Cable visited on holidays.

Maxine "helping" to trim a tree at The Gardens, 1999.

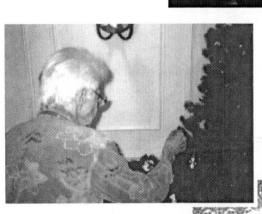

Opening Christmas presents at The Place in Tucson, 2002.

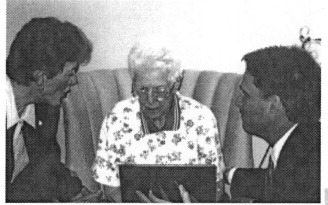

Bernie Freeman and Jeff Roley present a certificate to Max citing her academic achievements at the University of Illinois. Her response:"Want to touch me?"

With her favorite dish -- strawberry ice cream.

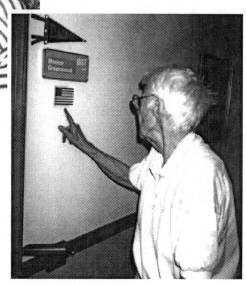

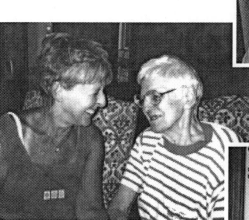

Jeanne Plant, Jim's daughter, and Max enjoy a good laugh.

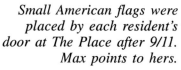

Small American flags were placed by each resident's door at The Place after 9/11. Max points to hers.

Portrait of Maxine that accompanied her obituary in several newspapers and on the Internet.

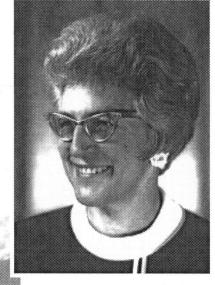

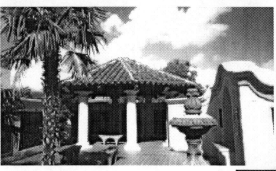

Valley Presbyterian Church in Green Valley, Arizona.

Church Columbarium, where Jim interred Maxine on their 33rd wedding anniversary, September 11, 2003.

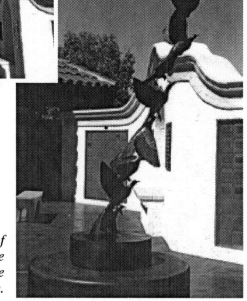

Lauri Slenning's bronze statue of doves ascending from the Columbarium, a spiritual tribute to those interred there.

CHAPTER 11

"Well, we haven't solved all the problems."

The search for Robin Henson's replacement, which began early in June 2000, finally ended with the hiring of Debby Shiflett in August of that year. Debby, a licensed practical nurse (LPN) with extensive healthcare administrative experience in the assisted living facility at La Posada, a Green Valley continuing care retirement community, came aboard as The Gardens' program director. And she faced a full plate of sticky issues that top management had been unable to resolve in a timely fashion.

I had already been in contact with Michael Hughes, regional director for The Fountains and the corporation's troubleshooter. I also met with Mary Jo Erickson in her front office. She was the executive director to whom The Gardens' staff reported during the interim between on-site directors. In fact, Mary Jo leaned heavily on Heather Hobbie for daily input. Heather was one of the "old hands" at the residence and Mary Jo relied on her objective reporting. The other caregivers seemed pleased with this arrangement.

It soon became obvious that such a temporary system of control, based on a loosely-linked chain of command, wasn't working. It was an inefficient, ineffective way to run things. Supervisors at The Inn, the assisted living component of The Fountains, oversaw their neighbors, The Gardens, assisted by Mary Jo's office. But it was not the same as having a dementia care manager on the premises.

Enter Debby Shiflett, who had the monumental task of winning the confidence and respect of her staff while playing catch-up with a plethora of operational records and overdue reports. She also learned that I wasn't the lone complainer. Gerri Sullivan, the daughter of Hazel "MiMi" Gillie, Maxine's first roommate, went on record with her concerns in a detailed, two-page letter to Michael Hughes. And she stated in it that her views represented those of five other "Gardens' families" as well.

When I selected The Gardens for my precious in 1998, it was the premier memory care residence in Tucson, if not in Arizona. In just two years, however, there were several drastic changes in key areas of dementia care management. Identifying these changes might forewarn other homes in the caregiving community that no matter how prudent and diligent managers may appear, inattention to some small detail or a belt-tightening in the wrong places could result in the loss of an institution's exemplary reputation.

Discussing negatives in a particular residence may assist families faced with placing a loved one in a new living situation. Selecting the right place is one of the most difficult decisions a family or individual can make in a lifetime. But by now, however, I'm confident The Gardens' management has corrected any deficiencies it may have incurred and the facility has once again regained its stature as one of the finest AD homes in the state.

In assessing the pros and cons of a residence, there are a few things family members must check repeatedly, such as the quality of the meals. Most people with Alzheimer's cannot handle food that is hard to eat, i.e., corn on the cob, overcooked meats, desserts filled with nuts, and so forth. Anyone in the advanced stages of Alzheimer's usually has difficulty in chewing and swallowing. They are prone to choke, which in itself is a problem without the aid of overdone, inappropriate foods.

One must be alert to staffing. The ratio of caregivers to residents should never drop below levels necessary to properly accommodate the needs of all residents. One and a half per six is the standard. Two per six is much better. To qualify for an Arizona certificate of competence in the personal service (caregiving) field, the applicant must complete a comprehensive classroom course of training, pass a written test, and demonstrate certain hands-on skills, including first aid and CPR. A felony record will deny employment.

Generally, the turnover rate among caregivers is rather high. Having said that, I should stress that caregivers are motivated more by their humanitarian instincts, than by financial reward. Yet, many have families and all are well aware of the fact their pay is usually not commensurate with their responsibilities. So, if a competing home offers them more money with everything else being equal, chances are they'll take the new job. And they will still get the personal satisfaction of helping victims of Alzheimer's.

There's an old expression that you can't tell a book by its cover. In weighing a care home for a loved one, be sure to look the place over very carefully. Poor housekeeping and poor property maintenance are difficult to hide. Check the condition of all the furnishings, the walls, the hallways, windows and trim. Flawed upkeep is easy to spot and speaks volumes about the quality of the overall operation.

As I indicated earlier, tracking medication is critical. In the summer of 2000, and unknown to me, Dr. Tenny Kentro prescribed Megace for Maxine to stimulate her appetite. When I confronted the doctor, he said he understood I had been informed. Actually, the medicine is an anti-estrogen commonly used to treat cancer. Among its side effects are constipation and myatrophy -- a weakness of the muscles. Maxine was experiencing both.

I also told the doctor I felt the drug Lasix was unnecessary. It had been prescribed following an examination of Maxine by one of the staff nurses. The nurse had detected "crackles" in Max's lower left lung lobe, which had been surgically removed in Wichita some 30 years before. A diuretic, the medicine was causing dizziness, dehydration and considerable discomfort. After the doctor reviewed Maxine's potassium levels, chest X-rays, and lab tests, he issued an order discontinuing both Magace and Lasix.

Occasionally, I received calls from a caregiver at night. Once I got one at midnight from Margaret Garcia informing me Maxine had fallen out of bed. She and Rebecca Blankenship found Max on the floor, tangled up in her walker. They examined her carefully and determined that Max had not been seriously hurt. Apparently Max didn't cry out when she fell, only when the caregivers put her back in bed. I had asked the staff to call me at any time -- day or night -- whenever anything out of the ordinary should happen to Max.

During this period, I noticed that caregiving in some areas had become lax. Several of the "old hands" had departed for other jobs in the local personal service industry. I still thought that the various issues I had discussed with management might be corrected in good time with the arrival of Debby Shiflett in the director's chair. I guess that was wishful thinking.

Maxine bruised easily and it showed, causing me to ferret out the sources. Some bruises could be traced to times she fell walking with her walker. Occasionally, whenever she appeared to be unsteady, the caregivers would wheel her to the dining room in a wheelchair. She wasn't too fond of wheelchairs, incidentally.

No matter what the mode of transit, however, it was the result of her performance at the table that counted. Happily, during the autumn weeks of 2000, she was eating better, much of it on her own. Whenever the caregivers saw Max turning away from her plate, one of them would sit down with her and try to get her to finish the meal. I did the same thing when I ate dinner with her. It took a lot of patience, but more often than not, she'd leave a "happy plate." And her weight bounced between 104 and 110, appreciably more than she had registered at the beginning of the year.

I always examined Maxine myself and one day she displayed some large bruises on both wrists. I asked the caregivers if they knew what may have caused them. It was a total mystery until Susan, the daughter of Ethel Jacobs, another resident, said she had seen a caregiver rush to get Max on her feet by grabbing both wrists and abruptly pulling her out of a chair. Caregivers don't mean to hurt anyone, but once in a while they might exert a little too much force in the handling of a resident.

Everyday I'd check Maxine's legs to see if she was wearing the T.E.D. anti-embolism stockings the doctors had prescribed for her. Occasionally she wasn't. The usual excuse was that her T.E.D.s had been misplaced, even though she had more than one pair. T.E.D. hose reduces the danger of thromboembolism by providing graduated compression from ankle to calf. But they must be worn daily.

A number of Maxine's teeth were broken, at least five of them, because of ice in her drink, whether it be water or a cold beverage of some kind. Caregivers and kitchen staff had been given specific instructions not to serve Max any liquid containing ice. But again, the message was not always communicated to a new hire. I'd see Max massaging the inside of her mouth and ask, "Does it hurt?" Maxine would reply, "No, but it doesn't look so good." And at times she was given to grinding her teeth, another sign of discomfort.

One day the caregivers and I noticed Max leaning to the left again and holding her left arm close to her side. She also dragged her left foot as she walked. I suggested to Heather Hobbie that it might have been another small stroke, not medication, that caused her inability to ambulate evenly. At my request, Dr. Kentro came to the residence and confirmed my suspicion after examining Maxine. He immediately ordered another CT scan.

The appointment was made at Northwest Hospital. Though I had arranged to take Max in The Gardens' van, which could handle a wheelchair, I was unable to get anyone to assist me because of a staff shortage. Once again I called on Robin Henson who graciously excused herself from her Sterling House duties and met me at the Outpatient Entrance. Robin helped me calm Max and lift her on a table in the CT-MRI lab. The technicians fully understood the problems associated with Alzheimer's patients and were every accommodating. Max did quite well, though the whole procedure frightened her.

A few days later, Dr. Kentro phoned me at home to report the results of the CT scan. He said there was no evidence of a major stroke, brain tumor or other anomaly. He added that Max had a little more fluid on her brain than normal, but not enough to require an invasive operation to remedy it. Naturally, I was much relieved and so informed Robin the next morning.

Interspersed with the most aggravating issues were a series of minor irritations, such as hunting for misplaced belongings, making up Maxine's room promptly and selecting her daily attire. On some days her blouses and pants were terribly mismatched. Maxine had always been very meticulous about her appearance.

Through all of this, Max continued to make pertinent and often timely remarks, indicating to me, at least, that she absorbed and understood some of the things going on around her. One day I tried hard to move her from the bed to a chair. Because of my diseased heart, I'm weight-limited as to what I can and cannot lift. I rang for help and caregiver Margarita Olarte responded. We took Max to the bathroom, but had great difficulty getting her properly seated on the commode. Max sized up the situation and said, with uncanny perception, "Well, we haven't solved all the problems."

Another time Rebecca Blankenship, the resident nurse, called me at home a little after 9 p.m. and advised me that Max had taken another tumble in her bedroom. "No need to come in," said Rebecca, "Maxine escaped the fall with a few scrapes and bruises, which I've already patched up." I arrived at 1:30 p.m. the next day and found Max still sitting in a wheelchair at a dining room table. She had eaten most of her lunch and was ready to move on. But she made it very clear that she wanted to use her walker, not somebody else's wheelchair.

Sitting together on one of the living room sofas, I reminded Maxine of all the ghostwriting I was doing for our good friend Jim Taylor, former Gates Learjet president who headed his own aviation management advisory service. (Until she became incapacitated with AD, she edited and typed the finished copy.) I said my articles, under Taylor's byline, appeared in several prominent aviation trade publications in the U.S. and abroad.

Ghostwriting is an honorable profession, I told Max, and I wish I had time to do more of it. "In the case of Jim Taylor," I said, "he gets the credit, or the blame, and we get the money." But I've been so busy lately, I added, I'm way behind in my billing for work I'd already performed. "Honey," Max said, "I wish you'd do better."

The summer of 2000 melted away with few additional surprises. John Wesley Adamson, one of the staff veterans, told me of a notation in the service book indicating Maxine had discharged some blood on her bottom. The night shift attributed it to hemorrhoids. I recalled that Max had her hemorrhoids surgically removed many years ago, but it's always possible they might return, unannounced. Anyway, that was the one and only time any bleeding from her anus had been reported.

I kept in touch with Robin, who generously volunteered to answer any question Debby Shiflett might have regarding residence operations. Debby appreciated the offer, but very candidly, was afraid her superiors would frown on her going to Robin for input. If true, it reflected management's attitude toward former employees. Either that or perhaps Debby didn't feel she needed any help.

However, had Debby talked with Robin, she might have avoided an issue that may have figured in her subsequent decision to quit her new job before she had settled in it. I guess I saw it coming. Though very solicitous in her relations with Maxine, even offering to care for her toenails and feet, which amounted to a free podiatry service, Debby's changing temperament mirrored her reactions to the pressures of a demanding position fraught with complexities.

Debby, a smart, intelligent, attractive lady, had been on the job a short time when, without advising me, moved a woman into MiMi's vacant side of Maxine's room. Ordinarily, this would have been fine but the woman, whom we'll call "Millie" to protect her privacy, had all the characteristics of someone with bipolar disorder, plus some of the worst behavioral patterns of Alzheimer's. Millie had been living alone, mainly because she didn't get along with anyone. At night she wandered, abused, and harassed the caregivers, and had virtually no hygienic discipline. Her bathroom was always a mess.

I confronted Debby, explaining that I had been told at the time I signed the contract for Maxine's care I'd be informed in advance of any contemplated change in resident pairing. Unfortunately, this policy was not spelled out in writing. Obviously, I said Millie's nature, attitude, and disposition were not compatible with Maxine's. She was loud, profane, disruptive.

Once again, I took my concerns to management -- specifically Michael Hughes and Mary Jo Erickson. And once again, both assured me corrective action would be taken, posthaste. After three weeks of meetings, negotiations, and interviews with caregivers, Dr. Jesse Pergrin was consulted for her opinion. After visiting the scene and talking with caregivers, she recommended Millie be moved out as soon as possible. The whole issue erupted because Debby needed Millie's room for a new male resident. He occupied it for a few days, before being rushed to the hospital, from which he never returned.

Arriving at The Gardens in the afternoon of September 27, 2000, Jennifer Richarte greeted me with the news that Max had fallen again trying to walk without her walker. She struck the wall with her head, causing a big, red lump. Debby examined the spot, then fixed a small icepack, which I held in place for about 20 minutes. Max, resting her head, said nothing else hurt. She did recall that something unusual had happened to her. But all she said about it was: "I guess I did something dumb."

As I tried to comfort Maxine, Millie, on the other side of the partition, kept babbling away and shouting for help. Several times she asked out loud who was talking on the other side of the room she shared with Max. Meanwhile, Mary Jo contacted me and said Millie would be moved back to her original room tomorrow, September 28. Next, Debby asked me if Lolla, a new resident, would be acceptable as Maxine's roommate. I had met Lolla and believed she and Maxine would get along famously. Lolla was gentle, kind, considerate, the direct opposite of Millie.

With the question of Maxine's roommate resolved at long last, I proceeded with plans to attend a symposium on the Pacific War at the Admiral Nimitz Foundation in Fredericksburg, Texas. Roxie met me at the Austin airport on September 29, and we motored there together for the two-day program.

As usual, I called The Gardens twice daily, happily learning that Max was doing well in my absence. Returning to Tucson at about noon on October 3, I drove directly to Casa Allegra at The Gardens. Jennifer met me with the astonishing news that Debby had abruptly resigned her position. While all the turmoil over the choice of Maxine's roommate may have influenced Debby's decision somewhat, I'm sure there were other contributing factors.

I felt bad about it and phoned Debby at home the next day, telling her I was surprised and disappointed to hear she had called it quits. She simply said the job she had held for less than two months got to be too much -- 10 to 14 hours a day, plus calls to her home at night for help with one problem or another. She added that she'd been "through all that before."

Though well-qualified professionally, Debby may have found the work at

Why?

The Gardens too stressful, compared with her managerial duties at La Posada. Indeed, pressures can quickly build up at a center for dementia care, as opposed to an assisted living facility. I mulled this over for a moment, then called Robin. "Guess what," I said, "we're back to square one!"

CHAPTER 12

"You better put me to sleep."

On October 6, 2000, I asked Mary Jo Erickson to contact D. Loren Wessel and reinstate his monthly podiatry service for Maxine. It had been suspended when Debby Shiflett offered to treat Max's feet at no charge. Mary Jo then said she had good news: "We've just hired Angela Ling to replace Debby." She added that Angela had been highly recommended by previous employers, one of whom was the Alterra Sterling House where Robin Henson had recently become that facility's newest director.

Angela Ling's academic credentials were very impressive. I had visions of Angela engaging Max in discussions about scholastic life on campus at their respective universities, or at least becoming well acquainted with Max because of their mutual interests in higher education. But, much to my surprise, the new director appeared too busy to develop any meaningful relationship with residents. She spent a lot of time in her pantry-size office, going back and forth between Casa Allegra and Casa Bonita, or "up on the hill" at high-level meetings in the executive suites.

But it was gratifying to know that management had moved swiftly in filling the director's empty chair. As to just how the new hire would work out, only time would tell. I'm sure all of the family members who had loved ones in residence at The Gardens were willing to give Angela Ling every chance.

For the next few weeks, my daily visits with Max were enjoyable and emotionally stimulating. She ate well for the most part, and appeared to be in reasonably good health. Melissa Skaggs, one of the more experienced caregivers, told me that when I walked past Maxine one day, Max said, "Now there's a man I'd like to have." Another time Max asked Mary to sit with her on the couch. But as she spotted me, Max told Mary to keep away and called me over. "Here," she said, "you sit with me." And every day when I'd ask Maxine if she'd like some ice cream, she'd say, "Of course!"

More than once I'd find Max's room in disarray, her bedspread, blankets and sheets pulled from the bed and some of her clothing piled in a heap. Finally I insisted the caregivers keep Maxine's door locked whenever she wasn't in the room. Seldom was anything actually missing, but at least one of the residents enjoyed prowling the building and moving things that weren't nailed down. Some residents were like little girls mischievously taunting their "elders" at every turn.

Max continued to complain about her tummy. Usually a purple pill (dicyclomine) relieved any cramping, but at times caregivers opted to give her a suppository, which generally cleared the bowels. I lunched with Max on her 84th birthday, October 20. The girls had decorated the dining room with colorful paper bunting and balloons. They also wrote a birthday message on the black-board and placed a "Happy Birthday" banner at the dining room entrance.

I think the significance of all the adulation registered with Max. She seemed pleased with the attention and the stack of B-day cards we went through several times over. Despite a light case of diarrhea, she ate all of her birthday cake and ice cream. I also met another potential roommate, Ida Ruth Davis, whom I had already approved based on interviews with her family and caregivers. As I got up to leave, it was music to my ears when Max said, "Jim, Jim, come here right now!"

Also that evening, I attended Angela Ling's first formal family council meeting at 6 p.m. She voiced some good ideas for improving The Gardens in a number of areas, but implementing them all or even individually would take considerable time and money. I told Angela not to be too disappointed if the bean counters turned her down due to the expense. I suggested she attach cost estimates for each plan if she could get someone in finance or maintenance to help her with the numbers. And I commended her for her diligence.

There were occasions when we couldn't get Maxine to adhere to protocol. Perhaps one of the reasons was that so many people were telling her what to do all the time. One afternoon at 4 p.m. the fire alarm rang for a practice evacuation of the two buildings. All the residents were escorted to the appropriate exits. All but Maxine. Dawn, one of the newer caregivers, said, "Maxine, the fire alarm is ringing, we must hurry and go." Max: "No, I'm not going. Take somebody else!"

Angela was trying hard to upgrade overall operations, but she always seemed rather distant. She was bright, resourceful, willing and energetic. After making a sincere effort to reduce the volume of paperwork, she finally reverted back to Robin Henson's system of record keeping. Some things can be a bit overwhelming.

As my former associates in business know, I'm a firm believer in flowers for the living. So I wrote a nice letter to Angela, in which I complimented her staff for their efforts in helping Maxine celebrate her 84th birthday. Angela promised to read the letter at the next staff meeting the following week. She didn't. So, I made copies and circulated them myself. The girls deserved credit for what they had done and I wanted them to know how much this old man appreciated it.

I sensed that corporate administration was still not totally responsive to the director's requests for support. My principal concern now oriented around staffing. Caregivers leaving their jobs at The Gardens were being replaced more often than not with contract people whose qualifications were questionable. Other staffers were working extra shifts because of scheduling irregularities. Working long hours continuously cannot help but take a terrible toll on a person both physically and mentally.

The high level of absenteeism and reliance on agency caregivers as opposed to full-fledged employees posed many internal problems. For one thing, contract staffers were not fully committed to their jobs. For another, as "temporary help" they never developed a good interactive relationship with residents. Some came in today, then were gone tomorrow.

I tried reminding myself not to become so obsessed with issues that I might lose sight of the real purpose of my daily visits with Maxine. I should keep my focus on lifting Maxine's spirits and bringing about a favorable impact on her quality of life. Also, I was having trouble with my own memory. I felt like the old man in a local retirement home. As the nurse walked by, he yelled, "Take it off!" "Take what off?" said the nurse. Old man: "I forget."

Maxine's health, comfort and care demanded my full attention, but operational problems bugged me. As in the case of running any kind of business or commercial enterprise, the core root of festering internal difficulties can usually be traced to a lack of effective communications. And if there's a breakdown anywhere along the line in the command chain, the net result can be catastrophic.

I spent my entire working life communicating -- first as a journalist, then as a public relations specialist and finally as an executive in industry and government service. The art and science of communications form the basis of successful negotiating, whether buying a new house, marketing a screenplay, rescuing hostages or planning the family's summer vacation.

My nephew, Michael Donaldson, is a successful attorney in the entertainment industry. He is an expert in the field of negotiation and has written several books on the subject. He sets limits, goals, and a point at which he'll back off if the negotiating exercise is beginning to wobble. Most important, he says, is preparation.

Negotiation is a corporate skill, just as is any other business discipline in the corporate culture. But dealing with management at Maxine's residence was a whole new experience for me. I've always thought my powers of persuasion could present a convincing argument for my position in virtually any contentious issue. Yet admittedly, I failed miserably in my efforts to correct certain grievances at The Gardens. Maybe it was a matter of semantics, relating to the meaning of language, or maybe nobody was really listening.

Anyway, all six of my girls (Maxine's three and my three) were well aware of my frustrations. Roxie phoned from Austin, Texas, and said she planned to spend Thanksgiving with us, which delighted me no end. I told her Maxine apppeared stable, though her disease did show signs of additional progression since Roxie saw her last.

I cautioned Roxie not to be surprised if Max was unable to say her name. Max doesn't always call me by name, usually substituting "you who" for Jim. I added that I often engaged in some therapeutic lying when I was getting ready to leave her. For instance, I'd say to Max, "Well Sweetheart, it's time for me to go back to the office." Sometimes she'd look at me quizically, as if I were making excuses to go. One afternoon I said I'd be back soon. Max rather sternly said, "How do you know I'll be here?"

At times I'd pause to reflect on the past and consider what, if anything, I might have done differently under the circumstances. Of course, neither of us had a clue as to the lousy hand we were going to be dealt. Benjamin Disraeli (1804-1881) put it well in a letter to Princess Louise on her engagement to the Marquess of Lorne, when he wrote, "There is no greater risk, perhaps, than matrimony, but there is nothing happier than a happy marriage."

I noted in my journal that when I arrived on October 28, 2000, Maxine appeared more agitated than usual. Seated in the foyer, she saw me coming, reached out and said, "You, who!" As we walked to her room, she talked in incomplete sentences. She repeatedly said, "Let's get going." Most of her re-marks, though, were unintelligible and disconnected, often an indication of a mild stroke or TIA. I tried to imagine what Max was trying to say and complete her thought. At one point she turned to me and said, "You better put me to sleep, I'm so disgusted."

Here we were in the twilight years of our life together, trying desperately to communicate with each other. I'd been married twice before; Maxine, once. The first time (1942-1946), I was young and naive and awash in the unpredictabilities of World War II. That union blessed me with a lovely daughter, Karen, born January 8, 1945. My second marriage (1947-1969) began unravel-ing early-on because of inevitable differences. I stuck it out until my two wonder-ful girls, Roxanne (born January 21, 1949), and Jeanne (born February 6, 1952), had reached maturity.

Maxine and I fell in love at Learjet. From the beginning, we both knew we wanted our relationship to last a lifetime. We had long conversations over the question of why our previous marriages hadn't worked out. Sure, we had differ-ences. Yet once we clearly understood how to "negotiate" successful together-ness, our loving consciousness kicked in toward all the ways we were unique. Consequently, we both determined to change the perception of any differences. The bottom line: we let our love go where it wanted to lead us.

As our adoration for each other grew stronger, it fostered an emotional, intellectual and spiritual evolution in each of us and in the intimacy of our relationship. It filled our hearts and souls with grace and humor. And in a practical sense, there never was a time in all the years of our marriage that we ever had a second thought about each other and our future together. Until we were struck by an incurable disease, we were inseparable.

As another Thanksgiving approached, I added some stories and jokes to my repertoire. Maxine especially liked anecdotes relating to our many trips, particu-larly our fishing expedition in Mexico. Naturally, I was given to some embellish-ment. I balanced my storytelling with readings from Max's favorite authors, such as Anne Morrow Lindbergh and Will Rogers. (We enjoyed visits with Will Rogers Jr. when he lived in nearby Tubac, Arizona.) Max also absorbed a lot of poetry while still able to read. Among her favorite poets were John Keats, Robert Browning, and Robert Frost. But she was especially fond of Emily Dickinson (1830-1886), whose concise lyrics, witty and aphoristic in style, were simple expressions, notable for their metrical variations.

I knew Roxie would be full of questions over the Thanksgiving holiday, so

I asked Angela if we might weigh Maxine once a week, instead of monthly. She agreed and drafted a memo to the staff, describing it as another personal service. I also told Angela that Max was complaining about a pain in her left ear. She had all the symptoms of a severe head cold.

Grace, The Fountains' nurse, checked Maxine and reported to Dr. Kentro, who prescribed Septin, an antibiotic to be taken twice daily for a period of 10 days. The drug did not replace the daily doses of her regular medication -- aspirin and folic acid. Max was also given a B-12 vitamin supplement on a monthly schedule. At one time we were considering either a heavier dose of B-12 or the same dosage more frequently, but it never happened.

A recent study showed that folic acid improves the memory of adults. Research also has proven that a diet higher in folate (a B vitamin found in grains and certain dark-colored fruits and vegetables) will help remedy a variety of diseases. Folate also lowers a woman's risk of bearing a child with serious birth defects of the brain and spinal cord. Some scientists suggest that it helps ward off heart disease and strokes, too. Others say Vitamin E pills won't prevent heart attacks.

Because of Maxine's advanced stage of Alzheimer's, all the new developments in research, no matter how promising, would have little positive benefit on her brain function. I made sure she drank plenty of liquids and always took her medication religiously. She started coughing again and complained that it made her chest hurt. Her left eye was drooping, but other than that, she appeared relatively normal.

I always tried to keep my precious pumped up, alternating between resting in her room and participating in selected Allegra activities. Her eating habits were generally fair and her weight remained constant, in the 105-pound range. On occasion, she walked without her walker, but the caregivers and I practically insisted that she use it regularly. Unfortunately, she had no recollection of ever falling when she walked without it.

Once again, I attended the USAF Thunderbirds Alumni Association biennial reunion in Las Vegas in mid-November, but stayed in close touch with The Gardens' staff while out of town. I returned in time for lunch with Max on November 20. The next day we sat on the couch, talking and reviewing her memory book, then walked to her room and laid down. On the bed, Max snuggled up, took my hand and kept repeating, "You're so good, I love you." If she only knew how much those words meant to me.

Roxie arrived the day before Thanksgiving and Maxine appeared happy to see her, though she asked Roxie's name repeatedly. The next day, November 23, we attended a delicious Thanksgiving dinner with all the trimmings at Allegra. Max, much to my delight, ate 100 percent of her meal -- turkey, ham, mashed potatoes, candied yams, dressing, greens, pumpkin soup, pumpkin pie, and fruit salad.

None of us in the dining room could believe all the food Max consumed. After Teresa pottied Maxine, we walked to her room and spent an hour or so just visiting. Roxie and I were both still full when I asked Maxine if she'd like to walk back to the dining room for some ice cream, although I had no idea where she might put it. Max didn't hesitate. She said, "Of course!"

Roxanne had long been fascinated by my "D.B. Cooper Story" and Maxine's role in helping me maintain close contact with FAA's "Com Center" (Command Center) during the only unsolved domestic skyjacking in U.S. history. It's an intriguing story and it had more than a casual impact on our lives. And the ultimate outcome of the whole dramatic episode remains a mystery to this day.

As we relaxed in Max's room, Roxie asked if I'd recall the details of that memorable Thanksgiving Eve in 1971. That was the night a nondescript man known only as D.B. Cooper parachuted from a Northwest Airlines 727 with $180,000 in $20 bills somewhere over the Pacific Northwest. (Cooper had specified $200,000 in his ransom note, but Northwest's CEO Donald Nyrop came up $20,000 short because of the difficulty obtaining so much cash on such short notice.) Cooper also requested four parachutes -- two chest chutes and two backpacks.

In those days, FAA had an anti-hijack task force composed of security, engineering, operations, communications, medical, and several other technical disciplines. Also in those days, we were averaging one or two acts of air piracy a week, mostly involving U.S. airlines. When we received word of a hijacking in progress, members of the team raced to the Com Center. Within minutes, we had an emergency radio telephone hookup with the FBI, CIA, ATC, State Department and White House situation room. We were also connected to the airline company and often the hijacked aircraft itself.

In the case of Cooper's crime, most of us on the anti-hijack team had left the FAA building. As is FAA's "after hours" policy, the Com Center reached us at home and patched everyone into a conference call with all the other entities. I urged Maxine to grab our telephone extension and quietly listen in on what I felt would be history in the making. Our system was guarded, but electronic eavesdropping was not uncommon.

FAA's purpose was to assess the situation, then recommend to the airline certain procedures that would ensure the safety of the passengers and crew. This is where Max came in. She continued to audit the dialog exchange for me in the event I had to leave my phone for whatever reason. As a result, Max was privy to critical conversations between the FAA, Captain William Scott, commander of the hijacked 727, Paul Soderlind, Northwest operations chief, and other key players linked to our network.

Due to my early experience with parachutes and parachuting, FAA Administrator Jack Shaffer named me as the team's "parachute expert." Asked why Cooper would want four parachutes, I said it may have been to "guarantee" his own safety. He wanted to make certain no one tampered with any of the chutes. Therefore, he gave us the impression he might force a crew member to select one of the chutes at random and then jump with him.

Cooper boarded Northwest Flight 305 in Portland, Oregon. Once airborne, he made his demands known to the crew. If they weren't met, he threatened to blow up the plane with a makeshift bomb he had in his possession. He collected the extortion money and parachutes during a brief stop in Seattle, where he released all 36 passengers and two flight attendants, Florence Schaffner and Alice Hancock. Next he ordered the remaining crew to fly to Mexico City.

Captain Scott told him they'd have to stop in Reno, Nevada, for fuel. Cooper agreed to the detour, but somewhere over the rugged mountain peaks on the way to Reno, he opened the tri-jet's rear airstair door at 10,000 feet and dove into the stormy night, money and all. He was wearing nothing more than a dark business suit, loafers, and a parachute. The outside temperature was seven degrees above zero, Fahrenheit.

Scott, his first officer Bill Rataczak, second officer Harold Anderson and flight attendant Tina Mucklow had a fair idea of the precise geographic position of their plane at the time D.B. Cooper bailed out. None believed he survived. Some of the loot, $5,800 in rotting $20 bills, and a tattered pilot chute, was recovered later from the Columbia River. But no other evidence of Cooper was ever found. And his fate is strictly speculation.

Cooper was the first sky pirate to "escape" by parachuting. Since then a number of others have tried emulating D.B., but all were either killed or captured. Today, all commercial airliners having aft exits are fitted with "Cooper Pins" to prevent the doors from being opened in flight.

Bill Scott rarely talked about the incident, leaving relations with the news media to his loquacious co-pilot, Bill Rataczak, who provided an entertaining cockpit view of aerial hijacking's boldest caper. But in retirement, Scott became less reticent, mainly to counter a public image of Cooper as some sort of legend or a "folk hero" who beat the system. In Scott's view, shared by most of us, Cooper was nothing more than a born loser who broke the law, big time. And he probably paid for it with his life.

Coincidentally, in 1993, much to our surprise, Scott and his wife Frances moved to Green Valley from Medicine Lake, Minnesota. We became reacquainted and, before he died in 2001, Scott spoke to the Aero Club of Arizona at our invitation. I asked Maxine what she thought of having Bill Scott suddenly appear in our backyard after some 22 years had passed since D.B. Cooper commandeered his airplane. She smiled, then said, "It really is a small world."

CHAPTER 13

"Well, for Heaven's sakes."

Christmas 2000 lacked the luster of the annual celebrations in previous years, though at times some caregivers and residents alike exuded an old-fashioned yuletide holiday spirit. With a little help from me, Maxine ate all of her rather sumptuous Christmas dinner, but she chipped yet another tooth because of ice in her drink, which I had not detected beforehand. Once again, I addressed the problem with caregivers and kitchen staff -- and the director.

All through the month of December, I tried sorting out all the pros and cons of keeping Max at The Gardens, or moving her to another residence. I'd met with Robin Henson and her boss, Lisa Jaramillo, to explore the possibility of transferring Maxine to the Alterra Sterling House, where Robin served as director. Both told me that if I wished to do so, they'd be happy to have her. In a technical sense, Sterling House was classified as a totallly secured "assisted living" facility. Some residents were still independent and cared for themselves, others suffered from dementia.

Continued use of contract personnel instead of house employees at The Gardens was an ill-advised solution for meeting staffing requirements. The Fountains, as the seat of power, should have insisted on a well-defined and promoted recruiting program. True, filling vacancies with temporary help is an expeditious way of dealing with the problem. It also obviates the need for training and other costly employee benefits.

Another major concern of mine was management's almost cavalier attitude toward the directed care service plan, the roadmap for resident caregiving.

Service plans are developed to indicate current levels of functional abilities and how the staff can meet specific goals in caregiving. Arizona's Department of Health requires a service plan review for families and/or representatives of each resident with AD every 90 days. Sadly, The Gardens' team had a lapse of memory when it came to complying with the state's prescribed review timetable, which I found unconscionable.

While I was 95 percent sure I'd relocate Maxine, the thought of Max being traumatized by the move delayed my final decision. In fact, I consulted a good friend, Dr. Don Griess, the "people's doctor," whose broad medical experience included geriatrics. I also spoke with Dr. Jessie Pergrin. Both said moving Max might be traumatic for me, but not for her. She'd handle it well.

I said nothing about my dilemma to any of the others at The Gardens, except a couple of the "old guard" caregivers in whom I had placed a great deal of trust. I did confirm to my family that I was seriously contemplating the move and the reasons why. I added that Sterling House was my first choice. It came as no surprise, as my three girls and Maxine's three had known of my frustrations in trying to get The Gardens back on its original track.

During the last six or eight weeks of the year 2000, Maxine did better than usual. She ate well, still weighed around 105 pounds and appeared generally cheerful. Earlier in the month she had all the signs of another cold. She also had difficulty in swallowing, which may have been due to one of her infrequent bouts with neuralgia. Whenever Max had neuralgic pains in her head, it almost always hurt her to swallow.

Dr. Tenny Kentro's associate, Dr. John Pifer, recommended no antibiotics this time. I told the caregivers to limit her to only one Tylenol at bedtime. I said, believe it or not, more than one a day will cause her confusion and an upset stomach.

At a Family Council meeting December 15, I told Mary Jo and Angela in front of the group that I still felt very uneasy in what I considered a worsening situation at The Gardens. The main issues in my mind, I said, were staffing, administrating, and communicating up and down the line. An example of the latter occured when Andy Colussy, the nurse in Dr. Kentro's office, visited Casa Allegra but did not see Maxine as instructed. She never got the word.

By now The Gardens' director and her superiors were well aware of my dissatisfaction. I was just as confident that no attempt to change my mind would ever be made by The Fountains hierarchy. And the more I thought about it, the more I believed Sterling House was a more value-based organization, incredibly committed to its mission. From my initial observation, Sterling House was always working on new processes and techniques. It focused on areas where resident care can and must be constantly improved.

My constant badgering of people in high places at The Fountains ricocheted down through the ranks. A new male resident was admitted to Casa Allegra despite behavioral problems which surfaced during his evaluation interview. (I'll name him "Henry" to mask his true identify.) Angela Ling kept a watchful eye on Henry until she had no other choice but to advise his family they had 30 days to relocate him to another facility.

Why? For several reasons: (1) Henry had been caught trying to crawl in bed with Maxine; (2) he kept approaching the other ladies and tried to fondle them; and (3) he made a pass at a new resident, who told him to go out and play in a busy street. Henry may have had AD, but nothing impeded his favorite sport -- womanizing.

The month was almost over when I finally got Angela to sit down with me and go over Maxine's service plan. It had been well over 90 days since the last one. I took exception to one grade -- continence. After a brief discussion, Angela agreed to reduce it from five to four. Max still had control over her bladder and, to some extent, her alimentary canal. But Max's colitis occasionally sparked her spastic colon with predictable results.

I had arranged to dine with Maxine and stay with her overnight December 31, 2000, the eve of the new millennium. I joined Max for supper, but she ate only about 50 percent of the meal due to some stomach pains. Caregiver Melissa Skaggs crushed a dicyclomine pill in Max's Equate supplement and between us we got her to drink it all. Referring to her tummy cramps, Max said, "I haven't had anything like this in a long time." At my suggestion, Melissa gave Max a suppository and presto -- action. Max had a good BM and her tummy ache disappeared almost immediately.

We were in bed at 8 p.m. and up at 10 for a potty trip and a change to a fresh pair of "fitted briefs," with Melissa's help. Max asked, "Where's Jim?" Back in bed, Max kept talking about a wide range of unrelated topics, seldom completing a whole sentence. At one point she took my hand and kissed it, and I kissed hers in return. Mary came in for a midnight check, then pottied Max again at 2:30 a.m., January 1, 2001. Max looked at me in bed and asked Mary who I was. "That's your husband Jim," said Mary. Max: "Well, for Heaven's sakes."

Mary got Maxine up again for another potty call. I arose at 7:30 a.m. and thoroughly surprised Renea Bond who had not been told (as requested) of my overnight stay with Max. The short staff carried a heavy load this morning, as several residents were in a high state of agitation. Margarite Olarte called Angela, who in turn asked Margaret Garcia to come in and help. Margaret had been off for New Year's Day.

Max ate most of her breakfast on our first day together of the new year -- and the new millennium (January 1, 2001). Nothing had been planned in the way of a New Year's Day observance and it was just as well. More agency people were filling in for absent staff, which family members had long been complaining about.

According to Mary, Max didn't get to bed that night until 3 a.m. the next morning, January 2. For some unexplained reason, she began crying, which was totally out of character for Maxine. Her tears kept flowing most of the morning, upsetting everyone on the staff. I called the girls (Marquita, Yvonne and Vivie), who were equally puzzled. They couldn't remember any instance when their mother sobbed, much less cried.

It was strictly a new phenomenon, one that was never repeated for as long as she lived. There were times, however, when she'd see me coming, Max might say, "Oh, I'm so happy I could cry!" And her eyes would become moist, though Max never actually cried, at least in front of me.

Despite the sudden, unexpected opening of Maxine's tear ducts, her general health remained stable during the early weeks of 2001. I'd already decided to move Max in February when I learned that Diana Will had been engaged to spend three weeks at The Gardens to review and correct any alleged deficiences. Her agreement with The Fountains included the possibility of a lucrative long-term contract to oversee The Gardens' two residences, Casa Allegra (A) and Casa Bonita (B).

I offered Diana my congratulations on her new role as the local institutional savior, though condolences might have been more fitting. She said she was well aware of my concerns and, in fact, expressed surprise I hadn't already moved Max. She suggested I might wait until she had a chance to work on the problems.

While I have the utmost respect for Diana's abilities, I told her my decision was cast in concrete. Later I learned that David Freshwater, CEO of Fountains Retirement Communities, Inc., which operated the company's far-flung facilities, accepted Diana's list of recommendations for certain operational changes, following her analysis of the major issues. In fact, Freshwater personally met with The Gardens' staff and reiterated his vision of making the two homes (A and B) the nation's number one center for memory care.

Encouraging words from the chief executive officer, but middle management failed to implement all the changes and Freshwater failed to follow through on his mandate for excellence. On the plus side, one of Diana Will's first administrative acts was the elimination of contract personnel, effective January 19, 2001.

A number of us applauded the action, but at the same time expressed some concern when told the regular staff would fill open slots while new hires were being processed. I cautioned Diana that some regular caregivers were already working 12, 14, even 16-hour shifts. I said it might be prudent to solicit their input, then develop a temporary schedule in concert with them, at least until the permanent staffing was employed and in place. But opposition to that idea was formidable.

Besides family members with loved ones in residence at Allegra or Bonita, I talked with individual caregivers, all of whom were equally concerned about existing conditions. John Wesley Adamson, for example, had transferred from another Fountains' property. He was frank and candid, but emotionally stressed out. The death of a resident always hit him hard.

Wesley reinforced my own observations: (1) the director had shown little interest in family needs; (2) there was no real direction, too many things were left undone; (3) agency people lacked compassion and feeling for the residents in their care; (4) only a few regular caregivers were sincerely interested in a resident's quality of life; and (5) The Gardens would do well to adopt the basic plans used so successfully in other like facilities in The Fountains nationwide network of senior communities.

Meanwhile, Maxine was eating fairly well and her weight still held at 105 pounds. Renea Bond often fed her and once said to Max, "Now if you don't eat the rest of your food, I'll spank you." Max feigned hurt in her facial expression, as if she was going to cry, then she'd burst out laughing. Renea said to me, "Maxine is so different when you're here. It's like she's trying hard to remember."

In the next few weeks, Max often ate 100 percent of her meals, many of them all by herself. However, caregivers were always ready to sit down and feed her if she appeared to vacillate at the dining room table. During the times I'd eat a meal with her, it was my total responsibility to help Max clean her plate.

On January 26, I placed a $250 deposit on a small apartment for Maxine at Alterra's Sterling House. I informed Diana Will, who didn't seem surprised. She had been making some progress in her multiple efforts to invoke administrative and operational changes, but admitted the daunting task was like pulling a truck uphill with a rope. Now that I was definitely moving, I wanted Diana to know that I had considered many factors. But it all boiled down to one fundamental justification: What's best for Maxine.

Lord knows, I've erred in judgment in the past, and no doubt will err again in the future. Yet moving my precious to another care home was based on a very thoughtful, careful analysis of the entire situation. And I factored in the knowledge I had gleaned from professionals in the healthcare field who were well acquainted with the circumstances leading up to my ultimate decision.

On February 16, the Family Council met with Laurie Pepper, senior vice president of The Fountains. Laurie also was now the executive director overseeing The Inn and The Gardens, replacing Mary Jo Erickson, who had been placed in charge of marketing and sales for the corporation. Angela Ling reported on staffing changes and emphasized that a full staff for The Gardens would be up and running by May. Angela added in front of Laurie and Mary Jo that she was experiencing some difficulty in getting responses to her requests for needed items and support.

The next day I joined Bernie Freeman for breakfast in Tucson. She was in town for the annual University of Illinois Foundation's special event luncheon at the Arizona Inn on Sunday, February 18. I briefed Bernie on my plans to move Maxine, then we drove to The Gardens to visit her. We met Max in the hallway and walked to her room. There Bernie showed Max pictures she had taken of Leal Elementary School in Urbana and the U of I's new H. Maxine Gladding Greenwood Video Editing Suite in the College of Communications.

At first Maxine didn't respond, she just looked curiously at Bernie. However, her face lit up as Bernie reminded her that Max had attended the Leal grade school in her hometown of Urbana. Max said to Bernie, "You're sweet." After the U of I luncheon the next day, Jeff Roley visited Maxine at The Gardens. And on February 19, 2001, I wrote -- and hand delivered -- the following letter, with show copies to David Freshwater, CEO of The Fountains, and Timothy Olcott, my estate and trust attorney:

February 19, 2001

Angela Ling, Program Director
The Gardens
5830 North Fountains Avenue
Tucson, Arizona 85704

Dear Angela:

I deeply regret that I must terminate my wife Maxine's residency at The Gardens within 30 days from this date. As Maxine's husband and power of attorney, I am not comfortable with all the administrative and program changes in recent months, and feel that my only viable option is relocation. I'll provide ample notice of the moving date and at that time will request medical records and other documents I might require, plus an accounting of any missing items.

My decision is in no way a reflection on the fine work of your core caregivers with whom I routinely interact as Maxine's spouse. The compassion and dedication they continue to exhibit in caring for my Maxine and other residents are outstanding examples of professional commitment. I've discussed my concerns with you and management a number of times and so far have seen little or no improvement in the issues I've raised, principally the lack of communication, lack of staffing continuity, and lack of individual resident activity.

A major concern is staff stress due to scheduling irregularities as well as the long hours employees log substituting for an unusually high level of absenteeism. Food service and the inadequate control over resident belongings have been among other complaints. As you well know, The Gardens was in noncompliance with the state-mandated 90-day service plan review, an infraction that I'm sure the Arizona Department of Health would find totally unacceptable. And I doubt if the corporate investors would tolerate it, either.

In my judgment, ever since last summer, The Fountains, by allowing economics to compromise its standards, even safety, has not acted in good faith, or in the best interest of residents. The dementia care market is very competitive. And anyone in it must be properly qualified, highly motivated, and fairly compensated. So, unless the company sets its house in order, it not only risks losing more good people, its problems today will become worse tomorrow.

Sincerely,

James R. Greenwood

David Freshwater responded on February 27, the day after we moved Maxine to the Alterra Sterling House. In his letter, copies of which went to Laurie Pepper, Mary Jo Erickson and Angela Ling, Freshwater thanked me for "the compliments about 'our core caregivers,'" whom , he said, have been called "Angels on Earth." He also thanked me for my "constructive criticism." And, he added, "we are constantly striving to improve our programs and your feedback will certainly help us do that."

Angela Ling did not answer in writing, but she met with me and spoke quite candidly about her own frustrations. She admitted she was "swimming upstream" with no real support from management. Angela also revealed she would try to effect some change in the short term, but whether she continued in place for the long term remained to be seen. "In all my working experience," said Angela, "I've never faced a situation like The Gardens."

CHAPTER 14

"Am I glad to see you!"

Monday, February 26, 2001 -- moving day. We planned to have Max at Sterling House in time for lunch, after which caregivers would keep her occupied until the movers had everything in place in her new apartment, number 807. The whole idea was to make the physical transition as simple as possible, with a minimum of disruption to Maxine's normal day. She'd see the differences between the two residences, perhaps, but nothing extreme and, in fact, the new accommodations might be a pleasant diversion. It projected that delightful element of newness.

Heather Hobbie and Melissa Skaggs, who were among the many caregivers who loved Maxine, helped me put her in my car for the three-mile drive to Sterling House. All the staff at Casa Allegra were sorry to see Max go, several of whom even shed a tear or two. Heather and Melissa were particularly touched when I took them both aside and thanked them profusely for being such caring friends.

Max seemed to enjoy the short car trip, commenting on the road signs, traffic, buildings, and landscape along the way. As I turned into the Sterling House driveway, I stopped the car. I wanted Max to see the single-story structure in its entirety. Its distinctive styling closely resembles a stately English manor house, with its native stone and white-sided exterior.

"Here we are, Sweetheart, this is our new home," I said. "It has all the appearance of a large, impressive mansion that belongs on someone's country estate or plantation. And dig that lawn," I continued, "you don't see many of those in southern Arizona." Then I watched her expression as she took it all in, hoping she'd make some appropriate remark. She did. She said, "Who cuts the grass?"

Robin Henson was there to meet us. Robin put her arms around Maxine and said, "I'm glad you came home." Max looked as if she recognized Robin from somewhere and gave her a big kiss. We were there in time for lunch; Maxine did especially well with her first meal in a strange dining room. She looked all around and said, "There are a lot of people here." I told her our new home was bigger, with a fine dining room that could accommodate all fifty residents at one sitting.

Following lunch, I left Maxine in the care of Stephanie Dyson while I exchanged "move-in" papers with Robin. We were also happy to see another old friend from The Gardens, Amy Voelkerding, who had recently joined the Sterling House staff. Robin had been accused of proselytizing employees from other facilities, but I was willing to testify to the fact that never happened.

Robin's staff introduced Maxine to the other residents and kept her busy while I returned to The Gardens. With the help of Frank Richarte (Jennifer's husband), I prepared everything for the movers. I'd hired Abrego Moving Systems, the outfit that had done such a great job for me before. In less than an hour, we had all the furnishings in the new apartment. Though small, it consisted of a bedroom, sitting room, and bathroom with a walk-in shower. It also featured a small kitchenette with all the necessary electrical appliances.

By the time I got back from taking Frank home, Robin had put away all of Maxine's belongings. Small photos were placed on her dresser and tables as before, and the larger pictures were arranged in proper position for hanging. Considering all the machinations I had weathered, culminating with the transfer, it's a wonder that I hadn't flipped out. I had dealt with a highly-diversified group of people. Reportedly, there is some good in everybody. But then, I haven't met everybody.

We came away from The Gardens without Maxine's last TB report, so Melissa "Missy" Townsend, nursing coordinator for Sterling House, introduced herself to Max, then injected her with a needle to get the required blood sample. Max had a few uncomplimentary things to say about the abrupt procedure with no advance warning.

Other staffers and several residents introduced themselves to Max, who was somewhat overwhelmed as the center of attention. Our first evening meal in our new dwelling consisted of onion soup, egg salad sandwich, sliced tomatoes, a soft drink, and lemon squares for dessert -- all among our supper favorites. Max and I were both tired, so Stephanie Tyson helped us get ready for bed. The whole staff knew that I had planned to stay with Max that first night to help her adjust to her new surroundings. Tiffany Glenn and Geri Hanson pottied Max at midnight and again at 3 a.m.

The girls got a kick out of Maxine's responses. As she was putting Max back to bed after her bathroom call, Tiffany said, "There, Maxine, isn't that better?" Max: "Almost." In the morning, Stephanie had a little trouble with Maxine's shoes. Max: "What are you doing?" Stephanie: "I'm trying to put your shoes on your feet, Maxine." Max: "Well you'd better learn how!"

Max ate very little of her first breakfast at Sterling House, but that was probably due to all the excitement of relocating the day before. I returned to The Gardens to pick up the small photos in Max's "memory box" on the wall outside her room. I'd forgotten them in the heat of the move. Kellie Wells asked Angela for the key to Max's box (each resident had a memory box, which was kept locked). After a brief search, they found it.

I gathered some needed supplies from our Green Valley home, such as glassware, dishes, utensils and the like, not for Maxine's use but to have available in case I wanted to fix something for our visitors. As Max watched me putting things away, I asked what she thought of her new apartment. "Yes," she said. "I was looking; it's pretty nice."

By the end of March it was fairly obvious that Maxine was as comfortable in her new residence as can be expected under the circumstances. She was eating better, though often with the help of a caregiver. Sterling House featured a spacious living room, TV room, beauty parlor, and another "sitting room" used as a chapel on Sundays for nondenominational services. My favorite (and Maxine's) was the old-fashioned ice cream parlor. Ice cream was available to all residents around the clock.

Robin said one morning when Max woke up she stretched out her arms and greeted Robin with, "Am I glad to see you!" Then they hugged and kissed like long-lost kin. Of course, there also were times when Robin would give Maxine instructions and Max would say, "No, I'm not going to do it, so there."

Within a few more weeks, Maxine's weight was up to 113 pounds. Her appetite had improved substantially and her general disposition seemed more cheerful. Another day, as Robin was feeding her ice cream, Max suddenly asked, "Where's that guy?" A moment later I approached. Robin said, "Here comes your hubby." Maxine replied, "He's a horse." I liked her euphemism. It was much more pleasant than if she had included the animal's rear end.

Robin and Mary Sivley, marketing office manager, both said Max appeared more alert now and seemed to be expressing her thoughts more clearly. But they qualified their observations by stressing that Alzheimer's progresses in only one direction -- it gets worse. And I shouldn't be misguided by any temporary signs of improvement in Maxine's demeanor or physical well-being.

In my brief exposure to Sterling so far, it appeared operations were well in hand and running smoothly. As I've mentioned before, resident activity was an area in which I was extremely interested. Holly Anderson, Sterling's life enrichment coordinator, had developed a wide range of programs she presented each weekday. They included games, contests, musical offerings, and special live performances by entertainers and speakers -- a little something for everyone. Even Max participated in certain activities, though she was never adverse to voicing her likes and dislikes.

Maxine seemed to enjoy walking to the dining room (with her walker), and sitting down at a table with other residents. Several of them, when they were with Max alone, tried to engage her in conversation. This was good. The best advice doctors can offer to slow the progression of Alzheimer's is exercising the brain. Max and other intellects like her always used their brains vigorously during their waking hours, ever since infancy.

One theory says that brains of the elderly segment of the population build up what's called a "cognitive reserve" during their lifetimes. Cognitive reserve is something you're born with. It's something that changes and can be modified over time. Today, the Alzheimer's Association sponsors free classes to teach people of any age, but especially baby boomers, just how to do it. They call it "Maintain Your Brain."

A brain weighs about two pounds, roughly the size of a cauliflower. Networks of blood vessels keep oxygen flowing to 100 billion brain cells. Branch-like tenacles extend from the ends of these cells, the brain's own special wiring to communicate. A healthy brain can continue to grow new neurons and rewire and adapt itself throughout old age.

I could tell Maxine's interaction with people aware of her condition, while they were still functioning normally, had introduced another dimension to her quality of life. If only the science of developing an individual's cognitive reserve had become available many years ago, it might have made a positive difference.

Just like your hearing and your vision, your brain changes with age. Doctors recommend you stay mentally active, increase the amount of blood flowing to the brain through exercise, stay curious and involved, and choose healthy foods. As far as I knew, Maxine, like many others, had done all of these things over the years and still fell victim to Alzheimer's. There are many things we do not understand about this dreaded disease despite the many advances in AD research. And that's why we're still asking why.

On March 14, Robin and Missy went over Maxine's service plan with me, explaining the grading system and the method of allocating so many points in each category, depending upon the level of assistance she required. It was similar to the plan used at The Gardens, but more comprehensive. I could easily detect Robin's fine hand in its format and content.

It was reassuring to see that the Sterling House environment, its ambiance, and the people, staff, and residents alike, were noticeably stimulating for Maxine. She was using her walker almost entirely, speaking to whomever was near, and spending quite a bit of time "hanging out" in Robin's office, especially if the director was there. One day, after Max devoured a cup of strawberry ice cream, we got on the bed and I tried singing a few of her favorite songs. She'd interrupt every other line. Then she said, "Now, I want you to get it, we need it." (Whatever "it" was.)

While I could repeat the same stories and jokes over and over again, I thought it best to increase my file of anecdotes about our many adventures together. For example, I remember vividly the huge number of Washington cocktail parties, receptions and dinners we political appointees were expected to attend.

The capital's social scene is generally busier than a hive of bees. It's where you pick up all sorts of timely gossip about government people in high places, some of which is true. If you're not present at these important events, chances are they'll be talking about you. Affairs like this, whether black tie or casual, is where long-established reputations can be enhanced or destroyed. It largely depends upon who's speaking to whom -- and the weight of the issues and persons being discussed.

Naturally, we enjoyed some gatherings more than others. Ed and Dottie Stimpson (he was president of the General Aviation Manufacturer Association), were among our more gracious hosts. As a Gates Learjet officer and FAA executive, I had frequent contact with Ed. I told Max he and Dottie were two of our favorite people. They even gave us the keys to their well-appointed hideaway cabin at the site of a famous Civil War fight near Fredericksburg, where we spent several delightful weekends amid a bevy of rare historic artifacts from the surrounding battlefield.

As the industry's pointman, Ed's efforts produced a steadily improving business environment for general aviation. He finished his distinguished career as U.S. ambassador to the International Civil Aviation Organization (ICAO), based in Montreal. Composed of 183 member countries, ICAO is an arm of the United Nations. It fosters development of international air transport by establishing a worldwide standard for procedures, safety, and navigation. As the voice of America, Ed proved to be a constructive force in resolving areas of disagreement in the ongoing deliberations.

The Stimpsons greatly admired and respected Maxine's views on controversial issues, though they may not have always agreed with her strong conservative position. Insightful, perceptive, Maxine advocated positive political change for the common good and deplored the social and sexual revolution that had been undermining our traditional family values since the 1960s. When the Stimpsons got word of Maxine's passing, Ed wrote, *"As usual, it was done with great style and class. What a lady."*

Another fun bash was hosted periodically by Wayne Parrish, founder and ruler of American Aviation Publications and his wife Frances Knight, director of the State Department's passport office, in their sumptuous Washington home. A distinctive feature prominent in the reception area was an exact replica of the symbol of Brussels, Belgium's capital, the unique Manneken Pis created by Frans Duqesnoy in the 17th century.

The lifelike statue of a naked little boy relieving himself in a small pond is fully "operational" using recycled water. It was rather startling to see for the first time, especially as a centerpiece inside the house, but the sculpture itself is a real work of art. Because of Maxine's abiding interest in all things artistic, I was anxious to get her initial reaction. "Well," she said, "to each his own."

That was in the early 1970s. Now we fast forward to 2001 and Sterling House. Imagine my surprise to learn that the owners of Alterra Healthcare were heavily in debt and on the brink of bankruptcy. Alterra continued to default on its payments to National Health Investors (NHI), which assumed control of Sterling House on April 1, 2001. NHI subsequently changed its name to The Place at Tucson. However, there were no other changes in policies, personnel, or operations.

Those of us with loved ones residing at The Place were told to make our rent and service charge payments directly to NHI, as it was now the entity in control. For several months, Milwaukee-based Alterra harassed us for the monies already paid to NHI. For me, its was more of a nuisance, since I had all the documents attesting to my timely payments of monthly fees.

The ultimate blow came when Alterra gave a collection agency its accounts receivable list and the authority to threaten us with a bad credit rating if we didn't pay up. I promptly contacted the State of Wisconsin's Department of Financial Institutions and sent them copies of all correspondence, cancelled checks and other supporting evidence refuting Alterra's allegations of delinquency. Other family members were in the same boat. Legally, NHI was the rightful owner. Two years later, Alterra filed to reorganize its other properties under Chapter 11 of the U.S. Bankruptcy Code.

I might inject here some useful financial data. Shortly before Maxine died, Dennis Scalpone, then director at The Place, offered a "capped rate" program for his facility's Directed Care, Personal Service Plan. This capped monthly rate included all of Max's personal and medical services provided by his staff and were not subject to change due to increases in her needs, which, in the course of a year, generally rose appreciably.

To me, the capped rate plan was most attractive. Maxine's base rate in July 2003 was $84.99 a day for the apartment, including laundry, housekeeping, and all meals. Her capped rate for personal and medical services was fixed at $27.01 for a daily total of $112.00. The base rate portion of the bill, of course, was subject to a cost-of-living increase annually, while personal and medical service charges remained frozen at $27.01.

Annualized, this worked out to about $40,880 a year. Added to that were prescription drugs, medical supplies, and the cost of all the incidentals and other items associated with Maxine's residency at The Place, bringing the total expense to around $50,000 a year. But under these circumstances, the cost of managed care is irrevelent, as long as you can afford it.

I recall that Maxine enjoyed her involvement in the business side of our marriage. In the days before AD, she handled all our finances -- the banking, purchases, and the monthly bills. We made investment decisions jointly and conservatively. Fortunately, we benefitted by liberal stock options at companies I had worked for, plus an accumulation of government savings bonds which remained salted away for that rainy day.

We were prudent in our spending, yet always satisfied our wants and needs. Both of us had been through some difficult times in our earlier years and now, besides securities, we focused on steadily adding to our savings account. As Cicero once wrote, "Frugality includes all the other virtues." And if I exposed my credit cards too often, Maxine would quote Ben Franklin, who said, "Beware of little expenses; a small leak will sink a great ship."

Max always balanced our checkbook and occasionally would ask me about an expenditure that I'd forgotten. Back then my powers of recall frequently failed me, causing both of us some concern. We knew little about Alzheimer's, other than it was a terrible disease that targeted the elderly. More recently, I came came across a report indicating simple memory tests can indicate up to 10 years in advance which seniors are likely to contract AD.

One such test required the subject to try and memorize a list of 15 words and repeat them back as many as possible after a short delay. The individual's performance was found to be closely linked to later incidences of the brain-destroying disease. According to geriatric research conducted at Toronto's Sunnybrook and Women's College Health Science Center, a normal recall for those ages 60 to 75 would be 10 or 11 words. Acceptable recall for those over 75 might be in the range of eight or nine words.

Because age and education are factored into the equation, researchers could not specify a precise point at which the numbers become worrisome. However, lower results in the range of four words could very well be a sign of problems to come. Had I known about this study when Max was 75, it might have been possible to arrive at a short-term prediction, roughly up to two years. As yet, no one has found such an early indicator.

Now my precious Maxine lived in a strange house, surrounded by strange people, including a strange man who called himself her husband, though she often called him her father. Life itself is all memory. It goes by so fast you may completely miss it. But if you have Alzheimer's, life is for the present instant.

Max had no retrospection. She knew not where she'd been, nor where she might be headed. She lived within herself, almost reclusively, despite the people and activity around her. That's why in the last few years of Maxine's life, I always thought of each minute of every hour we spent together as a truly magic moment, one to be treasured forever.

CHAPTER 15

"I want the best for you."

A good laugh is good for the heart and mind. Like exercise, it makes blood vessels work more efficiently, especially those in the brain. Laughter can ward off depression, one of the fundamental factors in the buildling blocks of dementia. It doesn't replace exercise, but laughing on a regular basis increases average blood flow 22 percent, while mental stress decreases it some 35 percent, according to studies developed by the American College of Cardiology.

That's one reason I was so determined to make Maxine laugh during my daily visits. Researchers have specifically looked at a tissue called endothelium, the lining of the vessels, including the ones so vital to the proper functioning of brain cells. The endothelium is the first line in the development of artheriosclerosis, better known as hardening of the arteries. It's conceiveable that laughing might be important to maintain a healthy endothelium, which not only could reduce the risk of cardiovascular disease, but delay the onset of depression leading to dementia.

Other scientists say the reason mentally and physically active people tend to have less Alzheimer's disease may be that education and exercise supercharge a broad set of genes involved in building a healthier brain. And laughing freely and often can stimulate genes involved in maintaining the health of neurons, constructing synoptic connections between them as new memories are laid down, and building arterial highways to supply more blood and nutrients to the brain. These are objects of ongoing studies at the University of Chicago and other research centers in the U.S.

Study findings are important because they have created a biological explanation for those very broad epidemiological observations about active lifestyle and education being related to less AD. And once again, much of what is being achieved in the research arena won't benefit persons already in the advanced stages of dementia, but the work is certainly deserving of generous public and private support.

Maxine and I were both great admirers of Art Linkletter, the longtime entertainer, writer, and motivational speaker. On a visit to the Learjet factory in Wichita, he inspired everyone with whom he came in contact. And on speaking engagements, at one time as often as four times a week, the affable octogenarian devoted much of his attention to supporting research aimed at understanding and curing Alzheimer's.

Author of *Old Age is Not for Sissies* and *Kids Say the Darnedest Things*, Linkletter, a straight-backed symbol of vigor and vitality, often jested about some of the Alzheimer's patients he'd met while traveling. Touring a home in St. Louis, he was introduced to one elderly woman. He asked, "Do you know who I am?" The lady said, "No, but if you go to the front desk, they'll tell you."

Linkletter has often said the two best interview subjects are children under 10 and people over 70. For the same reason -- they say the first thing that comes to mind. The children don't know what they're saying and the old folks don't care. Maxine was with me when my three-year-old great grandson, Shawn, looked at me, saw the deep creases around my mouth and chin, and suddenly said, "Granddaddy, you're face is broken."

I frequently told that amusing line to Max at her residence in Tucson. It was always new to her and brought a hearty laugh. As I've mentioned elsewhere, she had a great sense of humor and every so often, early in our marriage, Max related a brief story with a funny ending. For example, she once told of little Mary and her mother going next door for dinner. "Now Mary," said her mother, "if you clean your plate and Mrs. Brown invites you to have a second helping, you say, 'No thank you, I've had sufficiency so fanciful.'" Mary ate everything and Mrs. Brown asked if she wanted more. Mary said, "No thank you, my shimmy shirt and pants are full."

I often repeated the joke to Maxine and she laughed lustily as if she were hearing it for the first time. One rather lengthy quip with which I got a lot of mileage concerned little Johnny, who was filling in a big hole in his backyard. His nosy neighbor leaned over the fence and said, "Johnny, what on earth are you doing?" Johnny: "My pet goldfish died and I just buried him." Neighbor:

"That's an awful big hole for such a little fish." Johnny: "He's inside your cat."

One-liners were generally the most effective. People with AD can usually grasp short, punchy words more easily. Master of the snappy one-liners was the late Rodney Dangerfield. Examples: "I'm so ugly, when I was born the doctor slapped my mother."; "A girl phoned me the other day and said, 'Come on over, nobody's home.' I went over. Nobody was home."; "With my old man, I got no respect. I asked him, 'How can I get my kite in the air?' He told me to run off a cliff."

Perhaps the best source of short gags is *Milton Berle's Private Joke File* containing 10,000 of the world's funniest quips, anecdotes, and witticisms. Berle, whose career as one of America's greatest funnymen spanned more than half a century, gives a comical glance at such diverse subjects as business and honeymoons, lawyers and Avon ladies, doctors, and parrots. An encyclopedic reference for laughter, it includes selections from literally millions of jokes, both classic and those created by "Uncle Miltie" and his all-star team of comedy writers.

Maxine always laughed aloud at one of my favorite jokes not attributed to Berle or the Internet, even though it's longer than most I'd tell her. Church services were about to end one Sunday when Satan suddenly appeared in front of the altar. The pastor and all the parishioners quickly fled the premises in total fright. Only one elderly man in the last pew remained seated. Satan went to the man and asked, "Do you know who I am?" Old man: "Yes, of course!" Devil: "Then why aren't you as scared as everybody else?" Old man: "Because I've been married to your sister for over 60 years!"

I don't suggest that laughter is a substitute for exercise or any other activity designed to strengthen the lungs and muscles. On the other hand, if those who laugh on a regular basis are healthier, then there must be something to it, according to the University of Maryland School of Medicine.

Maryland's studies revealed that 30 minutes of exercise three times a week, and 15 minutes of laughter every day, are not only good for the vascular system, they can help ward off depression. As I've already pointed out, depression is a psychological disorder that can develop into dementia. Tests of heart failure patients who were also tested for depression have shown that those with mild depression had a 44 percent greater risk of dying. Also, depressed patients tend to make unhealthy lifestyle choices in such areas as diet and smoking.

Maxine enjoyed a healthy lifestyle, as family and friends will attest. For years we took morning walks together, anywhere from one to two miles. She didn't smoke and drank only socially. And Max pursued personal activities and relationships she felt enhanced the rhythm of her life. Also, she was conscious of the importance of a balanced diet. Even after I became the chief cook and bottle washer in our household, I did my best to maintain a daily program of proper nutrition.

Forgetful people often fail to eat well and, as a result, may suffer nutritional deficiencies. Sometimes this can make the symptoms of AD worse. That's why I exercised extreme care in the preparation of Maxine's breakfast, lunch, and dinner. When we dined out in the early stages of her dementia, I always ordered for her. I yielded to her only occasionally, such as granting her wishes for a Big Mac at McDonald's.

Visiting with Max day in and day out, I began noticing that she was having greater difficulty hearing me, unless I talked directly into one of her ears. At The Place, we had established a regular routine for removing earwax from both organs. But by mid-April 2001, Robin and Andy Colussy thought it best to discontinue further attempts to clean Maxine's ears as the procedure had become too frightening. "Stop it, stop it," Max would cry out. "I hate you!" The nurse and staff would continue to use eardrops at periodic intervals, however, which seemed to help.

One day I got on the subject of public speaking. As a matter of fact, I addressed the assisted living residents of The Place several times on such diverse topics as the Wright brothers, the illusionist David Copperfield, and my role in the Nixon administration. In the past, Max had always helped me hone my talks for content, grammar, and general interest. She'd often remind me that the speech, not the speaker, is what matters to an audience.

During my career, I've delivered scores of speeches, though always on subjects with which I was thoroughly familiar. When Max entered my life, the task of researching and preparing talks became much easier. As my editor, she insisted I spend time preparing my speeches with no pretense of spontaneity. Fortunately, I can read from a script in a manner that appears I am speaking from the heart or ad-libbing whole sections of my message.

Virtually every speech in the category of a "power house" contains at least one memorable phrase, such as "tear down this wall," "ask not," and "I have a dream." My talks about the Nixon days included a reference to members of the president's inner circle who got their "underwear caught in the Watergate wringer." For a number of years, "Watergate Wringer" was bantered about as being linked to misdeeds commited by the "president's men," one of whom was Bob Haldeman, White House chief of staff.

Haldeman caused me to be late for my own wedding, scheduled for 7 p.m., September 11, 1970, at the Old Presbyterian Meeting House in Alexandria, Virginia. Earlier that day, a Friday, my office had drafted a presidential statement detailing all the new countermeasures we had developed to prevent skyjacking. Nixon would announce them publicly the very next day.

For some inexplicable reason, Haldeman saw fit to hold up the president's final approval, which had been promised by 4 p.m. You can imagine my frustration as the senior man in charge of all FAA public information, especially presidential pronouncements related to civil aviation. I finally went to the White House and shook the copy loose -- without a single change in the narrative.

Whenever I revisited some significant experience with Maxine, I avoided getting into specifics. Her confused mind could only absorb so much detail. In this case, I simply said my late arrival at the church was due to a major project I had been working on all day for President Nixon. That seemed to be sufficient explanation, though it's unlikely she remembered anything about our wedding or even the fact we were married.

In light of subsequent events on our 31st wedding anniversary, September 11, 2001, it might be of interest to know what Nixon told America in 1970. He said FAA intended to place armed guards (sky marshals) on all U.S. airlines. We also would implement screening of all passengers and baggage at every commercial airport, as well as "security profiling" at every ticket counter and gate.

Once the spinal column of airline security, the profiling system proved its effectiveness time and again, as did FAA's legion of air marshals. Remember, in 1970, we were averaging one or two skyjackings a week, most of them involving U.S. carriers. As a direct result of the new countermeasures Nixon announced, FAA exposed a wide variety of lawbreakers at airport terminals -- fugitives, illegal aliens, smugglers, and other criminals.

For example, during the first six months of 1972, the first year we had all our deterrents in place, more than 189,800 travelers were identified as "selectees," or persons filling some aspect of FAA's profile. Of this total, 1,271 were denied boarding and 1,095 were arrested, more than half of them armed with some sort of concealed weapon. And many were carrying illicit drugs.

Regretably, profiling was soon labeled "discriminatory," an invasion of privacy, or an infringement of civil liberties. So, FAA's dominant security system was phased out under mounting pressures from various civil rights organizations, principally the ACLU (American Civil Liberties Union).

Had the 1970's system been operating, whether or not it would have prevented 9/11, is purely a matter of conjecture. Since then, of course, America's defenses against air piracy have been greatly improved, including the creation of a cabinet level Department of Homeland Security.

Maxine never knew that on our 31st anniversary, 19 terrorists hijacked four airline transports and crashed them into New York's Twin Towers, the Pentagon, and an open field in Pennsylvania after passengers thwarted an attempt to steer their stricken plane toward another federal building in Washington. Nor was she and the other residents with AD aware of a private plane crashing into a house the following Sunday within a few blocks of The Place. My reprise of 9/11 is only to put in proper perspective early efforts to combat terrorism despite news reports to the contrary.

I lunched with Maxine on our 31st anniversary. The girls had decorated our dining room table with brightly colored balloons. Adding to the festivities, the staff produced a special cake and joined the other residents in singing "Happy Anniversary." With a little help from me, Max ate everything on her plate. She talked all through the meal, making such comments as "let's go get my brother" and "we'll go home together." Robin had created a special card on her computer, signed by all the caregivers.

All through the summer I repeatedly checked Maxine's weight, which hovered between 108 and 111 pounds. She often fed herself, even though her stomach cramps were continually bothersome. It might have been my imagination, but it seemed to me the girls were giving Max suppositories more frequently now to bring on much-needed bowel movements. The girls denied increasing the treatment, however, saying it might have appeared so because of the higher rate of success in the bathroom.

We alternated the location of our visits inside The Place at Tucson, bouncing back and forth between dining room, living room, and apartment. When we walked to the apartment, I always pointed to Maxine's name plate just below the number 807. She'd study it, then ask where it came from. And I'd say everyone living at The Place had their name adjacent to their apartment number, which made it a lot easier for family and friends to find their loved ones.

Unless I served Max ice cream in 807, we'd walk to the ice cream parlor, pick out her favorite flavor (usually strawberry), and enjoy the old-fashioned atmosphere, as well as the frozen confection. By now Maxine was negotiating the halls almost exclusively with the aid of her walker. Also, I got the impression Max had become more talkative than usual. Most of her sentences were incomplete, but she couched much of what she had to say in terms of endearment, a real boost for my spirits.

At lunch one day, Maxine, sitting alone, spotted Robin on the other side of the dining room and called out, "You who, you who, can you help me?" Robin went over and fed Max the rest of her lunch. Near the end of her meal, Max said, "He'll be coming, I hope he'll be here." At that moment I arrived and sat down at her table.

"Surprise," I said. "I'm here!" Max then mumbled something about "this place, it's not nice. You can go now, you'll be much happier." I said, "No, I'm happiest when I'm with you." Max: "I want the best for you." I said, "I have the best -- you." Maxine grinned from ear to ear, leaned over and gave me a big kiss. And that really made my day.

Karen Kraus, my eldest daughter, flew out from Virginia for a short visit, her first since 1996. She expressed shock at seeing how much Maxine had deteriorated in five years. Actually, I didn't think Max had changed that much, but then, I was seeing her on a daily basis. Karen also commented on the way Max looked at me adoringly and kissed me frequently. She said Max certainly knew I belonged to her.

The next day Karen and I met Bill Lafferty for lunch, then we drove to Luke Air Force Base (just west of Phoenix), where I spoke to the local Daedalians at their dinner meeting. My son-in-law, Steve Sargeant (Vivie's husband) was commander of the 56th Fighter Wing based at Luke. Since then, he has served as deputy chief of staff of the coalition forces in Iraq and at this writing is an Air Force two-star (major general) on his third Korean assignment, this time as the deputy chief of staff, United Nations Command; United States Forces Korea.

As we moved toward the holiday season in the late autumn of 2001, Maxine remained in relatively good spirits, but my emotions needed some bolstering. I felt I was falling down on the job in some ways. My whole purpose in injecting humor into our daily "trysts" was to improve Maxine's well-being, the causes and consequences of which had a direct bearing on her happiness. Well-being and ill-being have a positive or negative effect on personal behavior, especially to someone with Alzheimer's.

Ed Diener, Alumni Distinguished Professor of Psychology at the University of Illinois, Urbana-Champaign, would become involved in the development of national indicators of life satisfaction, meaning, purpose, and engagement. While his studies and conclusions may not be applicable to those already burdened by AD, I was fascinated by the prospect of knowing how I, as an individual, might fit into the scheme of things.

All of which recalled something my mother said to me when I was a little boy --
and my response. It turned out to be one of the funniest quips in my stable of
jokes. And it never failed to evoke a good laugh whenever I repeated it to Maxine.
Mother said, "Jimmy, always remember, we were put here to help others." I
said, "And what were the others put here for?"

Other important research to be conducted at the U of I came along after
Maxine died, but it's something I wished had been available during my caregiving
days. It's call Healing the Mind Through the Life Cycle. Dean Joseph A. Flaherty
of the U of I's College of Medicine had charge of the program.

The studies would cover new discoveries in the fields of genetics, imaging,
and biochemistry, and the extraordinary impact of medicines used to treat
maladies such as anxiety, depression, AD, and other common afflictions of the
mind. University physicians and scientists are using exciting new techniques
and technologies to diagnose, treat, and hopefully, prevent these limited health
conditions that continue to strike so many people in our society, from childhood
through the senior years of life.

Speaking of genetics, recent studies at the University of Chicago provided
the first scientific evidence that the human brain is still evolving, a process that may
ultimately increase people's capacity to grow smarter. Two key brain-building
genes, which underwent dramatic changes in the past that coincided with huge
leaps in human intellectual development, are still undergoing rapid muta-
tions -- evolution's way of selecting new beneficial traits.

One of the mutated genes, called microcephalin, began its swift spread among
human ancestors about 37,000 years ago, preceding the historically productive
period marked by a creative explosion in music, art, religious expression, and
tool making. The other gene, ASPM (abnormal spindle-like microcephaly-
associated), arose only about 5,800 years ago, right around the time of writing
and the first civilization in Mesopotamia, which dates back to 7,000 BC.

While knowledge of the pressures on gene selection today come from an
increasingly complex and technologically-oriented society is intriguing and significant, I'd hope more attention -- and resources -- might be devoted to critical
medical needs here and now. Namely, more research into counter strategies for
slowing or stopping the debilitating effects of Alzheimer's.

I'm sure studies indicating a trend that's the defining characteristic of human
evolution -- the growth of brain size and complexity -- is essential science. But
I'm not so sure it is too important now to investigate a theory that our environment and the skills we need to survive in it are changing faster than we ever

imagined possible. There are many forces affecting our ability to withstand day-to-day existence. Certainly the contraction and progression of Alzheimer's is a leading one.

These new areas of scientific study will perhaps make an important contribution to the way we handle ourselves in the days ahead, yet some research findings are puzzling. Because of her higher intellect and general good health, and based on extensive study data accumulated to date, Maxine should have been among the last to contract Alzheimer's, if not escape the disease altogether.

With Thanksgiving coming, followed by Christmas, I debated whether I should do something special for my precious Maxine this year (2001). I finally decided to continue doing the other things that made her happy. There's no greater therapy than a good laugh. Humor can achieve contentment, happiness.

I told Max I wished one of our girls could make it over for Thanksgiving. I said how much we enjoyed having Roxanne with us last year. While Roxie was here we talked about participating in an FAA conference call during an actual aircraft hijacking. It reminded me, I said to Max, of Roxie's predilection for telephones when she was three years old. I was working at Hawthorne School of Aeronautics in Moultrie, Georgia, at the time.

Although I had mentioned the story of Roxie and her penchant for answering the phone, it always elicited a good laugh whenever I repeated it. Calls to our home were frequent on weekends, giving Roxie plenty of exercise racing to pick up the receiver before anyone else could reach it. Invariably, I'd be in the bathroom. And invariably, Roxie would tell the caller, "My daddy's on the potty, he's always on the potty!"

Humor based on fact is usually funnier than jokes made up. It's akin to the old parable, "truth is stranger than fiction." So if laughter is good for the heart and mind, it's also good for the soul. And as long as I could get Max to laugh at my corny jokes, I knew she was happy -- at least at that precise moment.

CHAPTER 16

"Is that so? I'll have to look it up."

Maxine came down with a severe cold a week before Thanksgiving 2001. She asked, "What's wrong with me?" I said, "I'm afraid you are catching cold." She said, "Can you help me?" I said, "I will, with the aid of our friends here." Max: "Oh, thank you." We were in her apartment. She was lying in bed when I arrived and needed to potty. I took her, then put her back in bed. She was heavily congested and running a fever.

Once again, the specter of pneumonia hovered over us. Robin had the caregivers keep Maxine in 807 after I left. I did get her to down a bowl of split pea soup and one of her favorite sandwiches -- peanut butter and jelly. She stayed in bed the next morning, too, but chose to sit up. Her eyes were swollen and very red underneath. In fact, the girls said they had to use a wet washcloth to open her eyes due to the amount of matter that had collected in and around them during the night.

Naturally, I was very worried. I explained Max's condition to Dr. Stanley Racz, my primary physician at the time. I told him Max had all the symptoms of flu -- she hadn't had her flu shot yet due to a shortage of vaccine. Racz gave me two vials of vaccine, which I turned over to Missy, the resident nurse at The Place. Also, Dr. Tenney Kentro prescribed five days of antibiotics starting the next day, November 20. I'm sure the good doctor could tell I was extremely concerned. Pneumonia and octogenarians are about as compatible as crocodiles and house cats.

Robin started Max on antibiotics, though she appeared somewhat improved, especially around the eyes. She was still coughing, but not so harshly as before. Robin also thought it wasn't necessary to give Max the medicines for breathing or allergies, which the doctor had prescribed for her earlier. Her breathing was normal and she had no abnormal reaction to sustenances or situations harmless to most people. Also, her flu shot would be delayed until Max had fully recovered from her chest cold.

We walked to the living room, sat on one of the divans, and I told Maxine she was looking much better. She responded by asking, "What's my name?" I said, "Maxine, Maxine Greenwood." She said, "That's right!" Then I told her Vivienne was coming to see us in a couple of days. Max said, "That's nice." I said she was driving here from Luke Air Force Base where her husband Steve serves as commander.

"No, she can't do that," said Max. "She doesn't know how." I said, "Well honey, you taught her to drive." Max: "No, I didn't teach her." When I finally left late that afternoon, I still hadn't convinced Vivie's mother that her youngest daughter was all grown up now and quite capable of safely operating her own car. In her mind's eye, Vivie was just a child.

Vivienne arrived the day before Thanksgiving for a five-hour visit. Max was feeling good -- and was in an exceptionally good mood. She appeared glad to see Vivie, who said, "Hi Mom, I'm Vivie, the youngest of your three daughters -- and your favorite." Maxine pondered the remark, then said, "One of them."

The three of us went directly to the library where Robin had arranged for us to have lunch with some degree of privacy. Max did well, eating most of her meal without help, which impressed Vivie. Back in 807 after lunch, or dinner as they referred to the noon meal, Max became quite talkative, though some of her sentences were incomplete. At times she was simply unable to finish her thought. Vivie turned to me, then back to Maxine, asking her mother, "Isn't he handsome?" Max: "Yes." Then Max looked at me and said, "You're beautiful, and I love you."

On that cheery note, Vivie left for the long drive back to Luke. I departed at suppertime and returned the next day for the annual Thanksgiving dinner. When I got there, I found James Henson, Robin's husband, reading to Max from a cruise magazine. Max was dressed in her new birthday outfit and looked stunning. She saw me and said loudly, "I love you." We thanked James for the reading and headed for the dining room. Max got the last serving of turkey as we were a little late. I had ham instead.

We walked to 807 and I gave Max a cup of ice cream, which she devoured as if it were the last ice cream on earth. I told Max it was good to see Vivienne again and the new nightgown she gave her mother was gorgeous. Max said, as if she disbelieved me, "Is that so? I'll have to look it up."

Over the next few days, Maxine continued to get better. Her weight was 108 and all her vital signs were in the normal range. While she seemed to have conquered whatever bug had bitten her, thanks to the antibiotics, I was feeling as if I might be coming down with something. In fact, I couldn't remember the last time I felt really good. I'd been on a fast track recently and some health issues were beginning to annoy me both mentally and physically.

I realized that when you reach a certain advanced age, the people who look and act the best are those who, over the years, have consistently eaten sensibly and exercised regularly. As the famous American poet and essayist Ralph Waldo Emerson commented, "The first wealth is health."

Most news accounts of poor health habits focus on the suffering and discomfort that people experience. But ill health can be costly in more ways than one. Compared with the rest of the population, sick people generally work (and earn) less, spend more on healthcare and have less time and energy to pursue goals. As a retiree with personal commitments oriented around my number one priority, Maxine, I may have been guilty of burning the candle at both ends. All too often I'd catch myself dozing off while driving home from The Place in the late afternoon or early evening.

Exhaustion, perhaps. But I simply couldn't afford to find myself in a situation that might escalate into something extremely serious. In other words, I suddenly realized I'd better invest in myself by maintaining good health. A major strategy is not to ignore small problems, but resolve them before they become major vexations. And I should see my doctor regularly and disclose any symptoms of what would portend larger complications.

Later I read a World Health Organization report indicating chronic ailments such as heart disease, cancer, and diabetes will kill nearly 400 million people over the next 10 years. Having experienced two heart attacks, a triple bypass, and a congestive heart that induced edema, such alarming information got my attention. The WHO study also found that prevention policies in Australia, the U.S., Canada, and England have helped cut heart disease death rates up to 70 percent in the last three decades.

Other than her disease and occasional colds, Maxine's general health remained fairly good. Her observations of the "good and the bad" were still there. One day I caught up with her in the library where Amy had taken her to look at some books. Max held a small, cardboard cabin in her hands. I said, "Isn't that a cute little house." She said, "I think it's dumb."

We walked to 807 and I got Max a cup of ice cream, prompting her to say, "This day is going well." Next I opened the pages of her U of I scrapbook and explained again the signficance of the pictures and stories and what had been done at the University to honor her memory.

I told Maxine that her Aunt Gladys had given her a box of three dainty hankies as a high school graduation present. I added that hidden between the cloth folds were three five-dollar bills. That $15 was exactly what she needed to pay for her first semester tuition at the University of Illinois. Max said, "That's right." I said the entry-level tuition today would probably run around $3,200 or more. Max: "Wow!"

Over the next few weeks, Maxine usually ate well, often on her own. But one December day, caregiver Terri Ruiz said she had "quite a time" feeding Max her dinner. Max kept chewing and chewing. Finally, Terri said, "Max, is your mouth full?" Max said, "I like you." Terri: "Come on Max, let's see what you have left." Max: "I like you a lot." Terri: "Open your mouth, Maxine." Max opened her mouth, smiling. She had one small piece of food she'd been chewing on. She said, "I'm full." And that was that.

The girls frequently said that caring for Maxine was a real joy -- full of funny surprises. They never knew what she was going to do or say. One day at the end of her shower, she started slipping and grabbed hold of one of Terri's breasts. She had a real strong grip, Terri recalled, but kept herself from falling.

In mid-December, I joined Harry Combs for a Learjet flight to Washington, D.C., and the Wright Brothers Memorial Trophy Dinner honoring Neil Armstrong. I'm glad I went. Besides Neil, I saw many other old friends -- Ed Stimpson, George Carneal, and Bob Anderson. Combs, Anderson, Lynn Krogh (head of International Jet Aviation, operators of Harry's Learjet), and I spent some time with Ken Hyde at his The Wright Brothers Experience facilities in Warrenton, Virginia, before returning to Arizona.

Ken had proposed that Harry fund an exact reproduction of the 1903 Wright Flyer, which he (Ken) would build and Combs would present to the National Park Service at the First Flight Centennial in Kitty Hawk on December 17, 2003. Harry agreed to do it, and asked me to handle all the contractual and administrative details with Hyde and the NPS. Consequently, I became deeply involved in much of the planning and staging of this 100th anniversary celebration commemorating history's first powered flight. A lot of work, but most rewarding.

While away, Robin and the other caregivers kept me informed of Maxine's condition via daily telephoning. Max still had a slight cough, but otherwise seemed to be doing well in my absence. Her appetite was fair and she continued to "entertain" the girls with her amusing remarks. Stephanie Dyson reported that she and Max had been talking about me. Stephanie said Max referred to me only as "he," not by my given name.

Arriving at The Place in the early afternoon of December 18, Robin said Max had fallen again last night. Third shift caregivers had found her on the floor at 12:30 a.m. She didn't appear to be hurt, but today she was leaning sharply to the left and her speech was slurred. Robin said Max had all the signs of another TIA (transient ischemic attack) or ministroke, similar to the ones she had suffered at The Gardens.

Under the circumstances, the staff elected to move Maxine in a wheelchair. Missy said she would talk with Dr. Kentro. In the meantime, I sat next to Max (on her right) in the TV room. She tried hard to pull herself close to me, but it was obviously too difficult. Yet she was very affectionate despite the TIA. Several times she told me she loved me. I responded with a hug and a kiss. Robin walked by and Max took her hand and kissed it.

The TIA had made Max quite listless and lethargic. For the next few days, caregivers coped with its lingering effects. Max was winding down another year with a slight cough and some imbalance, which would soon disappear. December 22 was observed as a "Snow Flake Fling," apparently an annual event at The Place. We sat with Vi Gallagher, Mary Sivley's mother, and Robin's parents, Bob and Janae Sharp. It was a fun evening. Max ate everything but her green beans -- and some decorative "snowflakes" under the glass tabletop, which she tried to pick up with her fork.

As the year 2001 neared its end, I reviewed the events that occurred since moving Max from The Gardens to The Place back on February 26. I was particularly pleased with the high quality of Robin's caregivers, but that didn't surprise me. I'd already sent my annual Christmas check to each of the staff, a practice I began at The Gardens. Sure, it was against corporate policy, but management, aware of my gifts, turned the other cheek (and even addressed the cards for me).

I've always believed in personally rewarding those employees of a residence whose job performance contributed much toward improving Maxine's quality of life. Over the past 10 months, I detected few glitches in operations at The Place -- each stumble was promptly corrected. Following are very brief verbatim excerpts gleaned from my daily journals covering the last seven days of 2001:

December 24 -- Christmas Eve. Arrived 3 p.m. Robin, Holly, Donie, Missy in Robin's office. Robin said Max "busy today." Max told her, "It hurts," and pointed to her rear end. Robin managed to get Max to release big BM, relieving the pain.

December 25 -- Christmas. Arrived at 11:30 a.m. Walked Max to dining room table, showed her two presents (gift wrapped). I said we'd go home and open them right after dinner. She seemed pleased and said, "All right." She was quite talkative, and eyed my coat and pants. So I said, "You picked out these clothes many years ago in a store in Wichita, Kansas." Max said, "I thought they looked good."

December 26 -- Called at 9:30 a.m. Mary Sively said Max still eating breakfast. Arrived at 2 p.m., electricity off at The Place. Showed Max new pictures of great grandchildren. About Jacob, one year old, Max said, "He's sweet." She also said Jennifer, two and a half, was "darling."

December 27 -- Called at 9:15 a.m.; Mary said Max ate all her breakfast and was in living room, ready for Holly Anderson's exercise period. Amy Voelkerding said to Max, "Here's your hubby Jim!" Max: "That's right." Vivie arrived (from Luke AFB) at 1:45 p.m. and said to her mother, "You're mighty pretty." Max: "You bet." Vivie talked across Max, who looked at me, winked and shook her head as if to say, "When is it my turn?"

December 28 -- Arrived at 1:15 p.m. Max in chair at northwest corner of living room. Pulled up another chair and sat beside her. We talked (I did most of the talking) about our adventures in Mexico and Europe. She seemed to enjoy stories, especially humorous anecdotes about our experiences traveling. (Note: Max had lost several pounds, but her weight today had returned to 108.)

December 29 -- Called 9:30 a.m. Terri said Max in good mood, ate all her breakfast. Arrived at 1:30 p.m.; Max in TV room, her sweater and pants badly soiled. Nichole said another resident gave Max chocolate ice cream, but couldn't identify her. "I didn't see her," said Nichole. Terri tried removing sweater but Max resisted. Max said, "No, it's mine!" She pulled away from Terri. I told Max to let me have the sweater so we could wash it. Then we'd put it back on her clean. Max let me take it off and give it to Terri for the washing machine. Max a bit fiesty today.

December 30 -- Called 9:30. Stephanie Dyson said Max ate good breakfast. Arrived 11:30. Max in TV room. We walked to her table in the dining room. She ate about 50 percent of her dinner. Kept spitting food out complaining of stomach cramps. We then walked to 807. Sat in chairs side by side and showed pictures of Vivie's visit, trip with Harry Combs to Washington. Max a bit anxious. I said, "We're home now, Sweetheart." She said, "I know it!"

December 31 -- New Year's Eve. Arrived 4 p.m. Max in TV room. Took her into dining room at 4:30 and we visited until meal was served. (Pizza, French onion soup, fruit, custard.) Max ate a little of each. Adam Huff also fixed her a peanut butter and jelly sandwich which she ate ravenously. I then walked her to 807 and put her to bed (time about 8 p.m.). After Nichole left, I got in bed. Max seemed to know I belonged there; she was all smiles and lovable. I helped her get settled, and for quite some time she held my hand.

Spending the night with Maxine on New Year's Eve had become a tradition ever since her AD forced us to live apart. There were times, however, when I seriously considered accepting Robin's offer to move in with Maxine in one of the larger apartments. Robin's figure of an additional $600 a month (including three meals a day) was quite an inducement. I finally dismissed the idea as not too practical, since I'd still be driving to and from Green Valley in order to take care of other business.

Last night was the best New Year's Eve ever. We saw the year 2002 come in together and Max never once asked who I was. She simply accepted me as someone who should be with her. In fact, she looked so pretty and so radiant, it was almost as if I was gazing at the Maxine I knew on our wedding day. That's the image I'd keep forever in my mind and heart. Nothing, not even the ravages of Alzheimer's, would ever erase it.

CHAPTER 17

"Okay, what comes next?"

Judy got Max up at 8 a.m. and prepared her for her first meal of the New Year. I told Max I couldn't stay for breakfast, because I needed to complete some work at the office. Maxine proceeded to interrogate me with all the fervor of a young attorney fresh out of law school. She insisted in knowing exactly what I had to do and why. I said it was a project for our good friend Harry Combs and it had to be done today. I promised to hurry. Max: "I hope so, you're gone a lot."

As I drove out of The Place's parking lot and turned west on Ina to reach Interstate 10, I wondered aloud -- why? Why did this happen to Maxine and not me? Was it part of the process of natural selection, or what? If healthy people, well-trained intellectually, are less likely to be stricken with Alzheimer's, why then did the disease target Max?

Maxine always ate sensibly, exercised regularly, and pursued a regimen of continuing education long after her formal schooling. It was a struggle, but ever since we were married, I got her to take an annual physical examination, expecially a mammogram. I firmly believe these yearly exams accounted for Maxine's generally good health. If the doctors saw anything amiss, they nipped it in the bud. Colitis was her only nemesis and we had learned to handle that. Indeed, Maxine did not fit the profile of someone who might become a victim of AD.

I headed south for Green Valley on I-10, my head filled with dozens of questions. I'd heard the drug industry was spending billions of dollars to come up with an effective memory pill, which I've discussed in an earlier chapter. So far nothing on the market can effectively improve thinking power and most treatments may cause a loss of appetite, nausea, and frequent bowel movements.

I previously mentioned memantine. It's no miracle cure, but clinical trials have demonstrated that the drug allows the most desperately confused patients to live independently for six months to a year longer than they would otherwise, with no debilitating side effects. But the big question in my mind: why has it taken so long for medical science to address this world problem? After all, Alzheimer's has been around for almost 100 years.

As I cruised along at 70, a speed I seldom ever exceeded, I also remembered reading that a cure for AD is unlikely at anytime in the near future. On the other hand, I also read that big advances were coming soon in the treatment and prevention of this fatal brain illness. Researchers have made big strides in learning about causes and possible therapies, and just in time too, according to the Alzheimer's Association, which stressed that the financial burden of the disease threatens to bankrupt our country's healthcare system.

I intercepted I-19 south and soon passed the turnoff for the mission San Xavier del Bac, one of the many historic shrines in southern Arizona Maxine and I enjoyed visiting, especially with out-of-town guests. Still thinking of the unanswered questions facing medical science, I caught myself slipping onto the highway shoulder. It was sort of a "wake-up call" for me to pay more attention to my driving.

Most of the technical details of Alzheimer's research are way over my head, but I was especially fascinated in learning something about the brain and how it works. Dr. James E. Crane says the mind stores an estimated 100 trillion bits of information. To arrive at such a conclusion, we must study memory systems, forms and types. Crane adds that various aspects of memory are manufactured by different biochemical procedures and are stored in different parts of the brain.

Although I'm getting ahead of my story, *Business Week* for September 1, 2003, offered a fine synopsis of how the brain's memory system operates. In an article titled "I Can't Remember," writer Catherine Arnst described brain function clearly and concisely. Here are some excerpts:

"The brain contains over a trillion neurons that constantly reconfigure themselves to form new memories or purge old ones. When everything is going right, they perform this task more efficiently than the world's fastest supercomputer. (Example) A phone number you've just heard is captured by the brain's cells, or neurons, as a pattern of electrical signals that transport it to a processing center deep inside the brain called the hippocampus, responsible for learning and memory.

"Once the phone number is lodged in the hippocampus, a cascade of brain chemicals called neurotransmitters is released. These messenger chemicals carry the information across tiny gaps, called synapses, connecting the neurons. The neurotransmitters deliver the phone number to the appropriate area of the brain for storage. The stronger the memory, the more synapses are created, strengthening the connections between neurons. Eventually a group of neurons band together to form a long-term storage space for the information, a process that can take hours or days."

My obsession with the brain led me to a study by a team of University of Southern California scientists who discovered that the brains of pathological liars, habitual cheats, and manipulators are structurally different from those of honest folks. Within a test group of 49 people, researchers found those known to be liars had up to 26 percent more pre-frontal white matter or wiring in the brain, and less prefrontal gray matter than others. Gray matter, brain cells connected by white matter, helps check the impulse to lie or cheat.

I mention this only to defuse any notion that therapeutic lying, a necessary technique in dealing with those afflicted with Alzheimer's, might be categorized as pathological lying. Not so. Whenever it came time for me to leave Maxine, I'd tell her the reason. I either had to go to my office or to an important meeting, but would return soon. And after leaving, if she asked caregivers where I'd gone, they'd tell her the same thing.

Actually, on every daily trip to The Place, my thoughts were constantly on Maxine and her care. I tried to think of ways I might do a better job. On this first day of 2002, as I turned off I-19 at Exit 65 and Esperanza Boulevard, I got a brilliant idea. At Abrego, I turned left again, then right on El Valle, just a half mile north from the intersection.

I pulled into my driveway at 435 El Valle, the last house on the street. It overlooks Haven Golf Course and the Santa Rita Mountains. I nursed my idea along and wondered why nobody had thought of it before. It was simply this: Certified caregivers are much in demand; they're in short supply, locally and nationally. And most young people who go into the healthcare field have little or no training. If they're lucky, they might land a job with a care management facility that trains new hires to provide basic personal care services to its residents.

It occurred to me that special homes for the sick, elderly, and disabled, including those with AD, would welcome a professional training center for aspiring caregivers. It would relieve them from the responsibility of in-house training and, at the same time, help resolve the critical shortage of qualified caregivers.

Soon as I got in the house, I made a few phone calls, only to learn that somebody else had beaten me to the punch. A nonprofit organization called the Direct Caregiver Association (DCA) was already planning a caregiver training center in collaboration with Goodwill Industries of Tucson.

The DCA had been launched in 2002, and was seeking funds for a new building through community development resources, potential employers, and private donations. Besides its core curriculum, the school trains people in stress management, time management, and communications. Direct caregivers are the healthcare workers who provide basic personal care. They bathe, feed, and dress patients, check their vital signs, and perform other tasks that can be done by someone with less training than a nurse.

Back at The Place, I told Robin about my idea, but somebody else had already thought of it. She was aware of DCA and its plans for a new training center. However, The Place would continue to train its own staff. Robin said her caregiver course was much more comprehensive and met standards higher than those required by the Arizona Department of Health Services.

The main reason DCA and Goodwill Industries merged is simply that the two agencies have a common goal for training workers who are underemployed and living on low incomes. It is expected that training school graduates would be able to find jobs with pay averaging more than $9.50 an hour, compared with the $5.50 an hour they were previously earning, on average.

Maxine was sitting just outside Robin's office, so I walked over and joined her. She was glad to see me. Stephanie reported that Max had been asking for me repeatedly ever since breakfast. I'd noticed that her eating, while generally good, had become more sporadic, whether it be breakfast, dinner, or supper. She varied from cleaning her plate to pushing her meal aside. Yet her weight so far had remained in the 108-pound range.

One morning Robin said Max was being ornery. In fact, for the first time, her behavior frustrated Terri, usually one of the most calm, even-tempered caregivers at The Place. Max kept spitting out her breakfast. Robin asked Max if she was being bad "just for fun." Max responded by spitting more scrambled eggs at Robin, laughing and saying, "I can if I want." Happily, she did much better at dinner that day. She didn't spit food at anybody.

Another day we sat talking in the TV room. Max suddenly said, "I don't know what I'm going to do." Again I said, "You're going to take care of me, Sweetheart, just like you've been doing." Her expression immediately changed from one of troubled concern to a real happy face. She beamed, her eyes sparkled, and she smiled broadly. She gave me a big kiss and said, "I love you."

Occasionally, not often, we'd have an "accident." I was helping Max with dinner, but she wasn't in the least bit hungry. Or so I thought. Actually, she complained of a stomach ache, a not-so-common occurence anymore. Brooke took Max to the potty in 807 and Amy examined her for a possible "impact" problem. But she had already started a BM, creating a huge mess. As Amy cleaned her up, Brooke changed her soiled panties for fresh briefs and slacks, moving Max to say, "Okay, what comes next?"

Driving the 35 miles to see Maxine every day gave me a chance to think of things I may not have already told her. For example, one of the highlights of our European trip in 1972, was visiting the Louvre, the historic Paris palace, mostly built during the reign of Louis XIV, now one of the world's largest and most famous art museums.

Our tour guide obviously was ill-informed about the Louvre's treasures, which include paintings by Rembrandt, Rubens, Titian, and Leonardo da Vinci, whose Mona Lisa is there. Other masterpieces in the collection are the painting in Gray and Black, known as "Whistler's Mother," and the Greek statues, the "Venus de Milo" and "Winged Victory." Members of our tour group quickly discovered their companion, Maxine, knew more about the artists and their work than our "highly-trained" French docent.

Max and I were also caught up in Western Americana. It's been said that our western heritage is the most unique cultural gift our country has to offer the rest of the world. We derived great pleasure in exposing historical myths and legends for what they really were.

According to Harry Oliver, for instance, the only way to learn anything about a lost gold mine is from just one man. If you go to two, what you know is cut in half. Go to three and you won't know anything. We motored all over the southwest, exploring old mining sites and ghost towns. We also followed the trails of such legendary outlaws as Frank and Jesse James, Butch Cassidy and the Sundance Kid, and the infamous Younger brothers -- Cole, Bob, and James.

While living in Kansas and then Arizona, we learned that Wyatt Earp, featured in books and television as the "west's most feared lawman," actually seldom wore a badge of any kind. In Wichita, he was not the sheriff, nor the marshal, nor the deputy to either of those lofty peacekeeping offices. He was just an ordinary constable and the owner of a prominent house of ill-repute.

Closer to home in Arizona, we'd visit western novelist Zane Grey's cabin in the high forest along the Mogollon Rim, north of Payson. Our mutual interest in western literature was stimulated by the fact that sales of Grey's prolific output were second only to *McGuffy's Reader* and the *Bible*. After 23 years, Grey left Arizona in a "huff" after his adopted state refused to grant him a hunting permit two weeks before bear season opened.

We also walked in the footsteps of Charles D. Poston, the so-called "Father of Arizona." A true pioneer of the region, he was instrumental in organizing it as a territory. In the 1850s, Poston was chief administrator of a silver mine near the historic settlement of Tubac, site of southern Arizona's first presidio. He said the area had "no law but love." Consequently, he assumed the authority to perform weddings, baptize children, and grant divorces. He also printed his own paper money for his employees long before Federal Reserve notes became standard instruments of exchange.

Dubbed "barnyard currency," the denomination on each Poston bill was represented not by a numeral, but by pictures of different animals so that the miners unable to read could determine the bill's value. The note featuring a rooster, for example, was worth 50 cents. Poston's "boletas" were accepted as legal tender at local stores in the mining district and in Mexico. And they could be redeemed for silver in San Francisco.

Though I'm sure she had no recollection of the incident, Max always seemed to get a kick out of my telling the story of our vacation with the Jim VanGilders on Elbow Key in the Bahamas. Jim, Mary Ann, Maxine and I piled into a small outboard motorboat for our first trip to town across the bay. I ran the engine wide open, but we didn't move an inch. Maxine noticed we were still tied to the dock and quietly suggested we remove the mooring line first, then try the motor.

As I told and re-told stories of our travels, many of them by backroads, I watched Maxine's expression. It changed little, except when I'd repeat a humorous anecdote involving some notorious character such as "Big Nose Kate," Doc Holiday's aging mistress. Through most of my storytelling, which I glamorized and romanticized, Max smiled politely. And she'd laugh out loud when I said something funny, such as the one about the sick cowboy who sent his horse for a doctor and it came back with a vet.

In our happier days, we'd occasionally do something offbeat just for kicks. Maxine had heard about a color specialist, Rebecca Hume, who tested people to determine their personality by colors. I accidentally found the results of Max's test, taken November 28, 1987, in Tucson. When I read the report to her, she smiled and said, "Interesting." Here's how Max was described:

"You are rather a showoff at times. Often you feel bright and cheery but cannot express it. Life is a joy to you. Like jewels, you seek wealth in the friendship of others. All life surrounds you in infinite joy. Self-assured on the outside, you sometimes doubt your choices. Your home, like you, is dramatic and striking. A fear of being thought gaudy, you downplay a more colorful nature."

The complete "Composite Personality" section of the analysis is rather lengthy, so I'll simply quote the lead item: "Your color choices place you in the category of a Striking Spring, meaning that your personality is dominate in the Spring (Sanguine) temperment type, and are blended with Winter (Melancholic)."

Surprisingly, the full report hit the mark in many areas -- all on the positive side. I think Max wanted to ask me about mine, but I headed her off by saying I hadn't come across it yet. From her expression, she figured I didn't like the results. Actually, the fact I didn't have mine immediately at hand was the simple truth. And I'm still looking for it, though finding it now is no longer important.

During the first half of 2002, Max was occasionally agitated and irritable. She also lost her glasses every now and then, even after we attached them to a safety strap, which she managed to disengage. I also noticed Maxine tiring more and becoming winded as we walked from one area to another in The Place, usually with the aid of a walker. I realized this was to be expected, but it still worried me.

Max also picked up an annoying habit by mid-year. She began pounding on the dining room table to get attention. Her noisy calls for service so upset her nearby neighbors that Robin had to move Max to another table. But my biggest concern at this point was her total lack of stamina. Whenever she became a little antsy, she was tired.

I also observed that Max was rubbing her gums with her fingers more frequently now. I told Robin to have the staff check for any sign of pain inside or around Maxine's mouth. Her teeth were in bad shape, but seeing a dentist wasn't really a viable option at this time. Perhaps later, if the pain persisted.

Though there were clear signs of physical deterioration, Max's continued ability to talk, even in broken sentences, gave me some encouragement. Here's an exchange that occurred at dinner one day when I had to blow my nose. Max: "Did you get it all out?" Next, she asked about the food in front of us. I said,

Why?

"It's our dinner." Max: "That's what I'd call it."

Terri and I took Max to 807 and her potty, then Max and I laid down together on her bed. Max said, "Now, don't go away, at least for a little bit." Then she added, "I don't want to be doing goofy things." She patted her tummy and said, "For some reason, they put something in here. I don't know what it is." I said, "I'll find out, Sweetheart." Max: "I hope you can." Obviously she was having another bout with stomach cramps.

As the weeks and months rolled by, I continued to look for more physical signs of the disease's progression. I'm sure they were there, but being so close to Max on a daily basis, I might have missed something right under my nose. Her hearing was worse, some teeth bothered her and walking had become much more difficult.

Ever since Max was diagnosed with Alzheimer's in 1990, I read numerous books and papers on the disease and how best to care for a loved one who had it. One book I found most helpful was titled *Alzheimer's: A Caregivers Guide and Source Book* by Howard Gruetzner, published in 1988 by John Wiley & Sons, Inc. I referred to it frequently. And now, with Max on the so-called last level of AD, the following paragraph is most pertinent:

"Such phrases as 'a long good-bye' or an 'unending death' have been used to describe the disease's final stage. Caregivers must give so much for so small a response that often all the questions of life seem to be best summed up in one word -- 'Why?'"

I asked myself repeatedly, was I really prepared for the inevitable? As author Guetzner wrote, the AD victim's "motor abilities will continue to deteriorate and eventually the ability to walk, sit, and smile will be lost, as well as control of bladder and colon functions." The mere thought of life without Maxine, even in her impaired state, was almost too much for me to contemplate. She was my living, breathing precious and I felt the warmth of her love and devotion whenever we were together.

When I'd tell Max that I was going to take care of her just like she took care of me for so many years, she'd smile and say, "That's good!" One day Max really sparkled when I told her we'd just finished a lot of work. "What was it?" she asked. I showed her the drafts of four biographical sketches of the nominees who were to be enshrined in the Arizona Aviation Hall of Fame. I said she'd helped me with some writing, did all the editing, and made some great suggestions for improving my prose. She seemed real pleased to have been part of an active project.

It's important to help an individual with AD to walk as long as possible. The use of geriatric chairs and other like devices should be avoided unless absolutely necessary. Such confinement increases agitation and restlessness. Maxine, as I've said, didn't even like wheelchairs. Once, as I was helping Norma Anderson seat Max in hers, she said, rather angrily, "What are you doing?" Norma: "I'm taking you to the potty." Max pointing at me said, "Take him first!"

I also knew that there would be a point in Maxine's final stage where she'd lose the ability to chew and swallow food. The dietician, of course, would prepare only soft foods for her and, ultimately would puree everything. And as time went on, Max's vulnerability to seizures, aspirations, pneumonia and other illnesses would increase.

During the second half of 2002, Maxine fell several times at night in her apartment, fortunately without seriously hurting herself. One time caregivers found her asleep on the bathroom floor. She had a large bump on her nose, but otherwise came through the nocturnal mishap relatively unscathed.

At summer's end, Robin and I took Maxine to a highly-recommended oral surgeon for a complete dental examination. It seemed to us that her teeth were causing Max more discomfort than she would admit. At the conclusion of the his exam, the doctor said all four broken teeth should be pulled at once. This would involve a heavy dose of an anesthetic and post-operative care largely administered by the patient -- Maxine. Aside from the trauma, Max would never be able to hold a mouthful of gauze long enough for the gums to heal.

After weighing all the pros and cons, Robin and I decided to pass on the proposed operation and treat Maxine's teeth problems with painkillers and other medication. Extracting the teeth was the best solution, but to do four at once would be much too hard on Max and the doctor refused to consider taking them out one at a time over a period of two weeks.

Thanksgiving Day 2002 (November 28) was rather low key, none of the girls could join us. Rachael Stevenson helped me transport Maxine to the dining room, partly via her walker, but mostly in a wheelchair after she slumped down. We never could get Max to place her feet on the wheelchair's foot plates, so we always had to pull her backwards. Otherwise her feet would drag on the floor. When we moved her, Max could see where she'd been, but not where she was going. We made a guessing game out of it.

The traditional turkey dinner this Thanksgiving Day was excellent, and Maxine was in good spirits. During the meal (Max ate most of it), I reflected on the years of our life together. They were happy years. From the day of our wedding, we found harmony within ourselves. As an old wise man once said, "An inner balance makes it possible to act from reason rather than emotion." How true.

We finished dinner and moved from the table to a sofa in the living room. "You are my sweetheart," said Max as we sat down. I said, "And you are my precious." Max: "That's what I've been telling you." I showed her Vivie's Thanksgiving Day card and said I'd put it away with the others. Max: "Yes, I got quite a lot." I walked to 807, placed the card in Maxine's top dresser drawer, glanced at all the photos which triggered a host of fond memories, and returned to the sofa.

"May I sit here with you," I asked. Max: "Yes, but be a good boy." Then she put her arm around me and said, "You do things right and I love you." I kissed her on the lips. Suddenly, all our troubles vanished from my mind as I kissed her again. And I thought to myself, I really do have a lot to be thankful for.

CHAPTER 18

"Not good!"

I ended the year 2002 by spending both Christmas Eve and New Year's Eve with my precious. As the holidays approached, Maxine appeared to be in good spirits, but her coordination continued to worsen. Also, she required the use of a wheelchair more frequently. Her weight fluctuated between 105 and 112 pounds, largely depending on how well she was eating. Even though she might eat poorly, however, she always drank her strawberry Equate supplement.

The week before Christmas was fairly active. At times, Maxine would be seated with another resident, Rosella, who talked her ears off. Max didn't understand anything Rosella said, but she listened patiently. When I arrived on the scene one day, Debra Reid moved Rosella from the sofa to a chair, so I could sit next to Max and show her the Christmas cards she received from the girls. Her reaction: "Oh gosh!"

We were now seating Max at the dining room table in her wheelchair, not the most comfortable arrangement but it was easier for the caregivers. After feeding Max dinner on December 22, Michele and I wheeled Max to 807 and the potty. (Michelle had to call Debra to help get Max unstuck from the toilet.) We laid down for a rest and at 3:30 p.m. I asked Max if she wanted to get up. She said, "Yes, but I don't know why."

The next day I scolded Robin for not staying home. She was still suffering from a bad case of bronchitis. Moreover, she was going outside to smoke in 40-degree weather without a coat. Inside, Max was enjoying one of Holly Anderson's musical programs, the Tucson Ringers (an English handbell group). Max was sitting in her wheelchair, clapping away. When the ringers stopped ringing to talk, Max said, "Go ahead," implying they should keep ringing and stop talking.

I arrived at 4 p.m., December 24, for a great Christmas Eve with my beloved Maxine. For supper, George Ojeda told Max the kitchen had fixed her a peanut butter and jelly sandwich instead of the bologna on the menu. "You like peanut butter and jelly, don't you Max?" George asked. Max: "Oh, yes!" I cut in and said, "This is Christmas Eve, Santa Claus is coming." Max: "That's crazy!"

When I told her we'd been together more than 35 years, Max replied, "Oh for goodness sake." While eating our Christmas Eve supper, Max suddenly said, "Do you think you're going to be loyal?" I said, "Loyal to you, of course!" I added, "Weve got a lot to talk about tonight." Max: "Yes, I know."

We were in bed by 8 p.m., both of us quite sleepy. It was obvious any conversation we planned would have to be deferred or postponed. Rachael Stevenson (3rd shift) came in at 11 p.m., then 1, 4 and 6 a.m. to check and potty Max. After midnight, before Rachael got Max up at 1 a.m., I told Max it was Christmas Day. Thirty minutes later, as Max sat on the potty, she looked up at Rachael and, right out of the blue, said, "Christmas!"

I remained with Max until suppertime Christmas Day, then I reluctantly departed. But being with her for 24 hours straight made it the best Christmas I'd had in many years. In bed, Max put her arm around me (and didn't even ask who I was) and held my hand tightly. In fact, she wouldn't let go when I had to get up and go to the bathroom.

New Year's Eve I arrived in time for supper, which Max ate in its entirety, including her usual supplement. About the meal, Max said, "This is good." About the evening musical (Jack and Nancy Roach), "This is awful!" Actually, it was quite entertaining. Because of her hearing defect, Max critiqued programs as either "too loud" or "can't hear you."

Once again we were in bed by 8 p.m. Then Kelly (3rd shift) came and took Maxine to the bathroom at 12:45 a.m. I said to Max, "Guess what, Sweetheart, we're beginning a new year. It's the first day of 2003!" Max, virtually emotionless, said, "Hooray."

After breakfast, Gina pottied Max in 807. We stayed in the apartment throughout the morning. I explained to my precious the significance of the year 2003 to the aviation community. (It marked the 100th anniversary of history's first successful powered airplane flight.) I also showed Max her copy of *Kill Devil Hill: Discovering the Secret of the Wright Brothers* (by Harry Combs) and explained her vital role in the book's production. Then I sang several of her favorite songs, after which I remarked, "I sure wish I could sing." Max: "So do I."

During the next few weeks, Maxine ate fairly well and hardly complained about her stomach and teeth. Whenever she mentioned a toothache, the caregivers applied pain-relieving Orajel on the gums around the affected tooth. And on March 31, just when I thought Max was doing so well, Robin called me at 1 p.m. to tell me they were taking Max by ambulance to Northwest Medical Center's Emergency Room. She was suspected of having pneumonia.

Fearing the worst, I rushed to the hospital at speeds well above my self-imposed 70 miles-per-hour limit, arriving at the ER entrance at 1:35 p.m. A Dr. Nannin had already ordered chest X-rays, blood tests and a urine specimen. His immediate evaluation indicated a lung infection. Robin said that at lunch Maxine acted as if she was having a seizure. The doctor put Max on oxygen and gave her antibiotics intravenously. Her blood pressure was high and her temperature, 101.

By 10 p.m. we had Max settled in Room 376. I stayed with her overnight. By morning her blood pressure and temperature were back in normal range. Max slept well, but I didn't. The small folding cot they gave me was more like a medieval, sleep-depriving torture rack. They should offer back therapy with every cot.

Dr. Tenney Kentro saw Max daily until he released her. I spent every morning and afternoon with her, usually helping with her meals. On April 3, Max awoke when she heard me enter the room. I greeted her and Max said, "I love you." Then she added, "I can't come out and play now." (Another childhood retrogression.)

Kentro came in at noon, checked Max from head to toe, then asked her if she'd like to go home today. Max: "Let's go now!" In retrospect, I must say the care Max received at Northwest was outstanding. She was a mighty sick lady when admitted, but the doctors and nurses cured her in a little over 72 hours. And she was happy to be "home," though her comments about my driving the short distance from the hospital won't be repeated here.

April was an eventful month; some surprises, some disappointments. After giving Robin all the hospital's paperwork, she knocked me over with the news she'd be leaving soon to join her sister's company in Tempe, Arizona. It's called TOLT Service Group and Tammy Brown, Robin's sister, is senior vice president and company founder. TOLT stands for Team One Logistics and Technology. It provides computer maintenance services to major retail shopping chains and other businesses, nationwide.

While I hated to see Robin leave, I realized TOLT offered her greater opportunity for growth -- professionally and financially. Besides her superior capabilities in healthcare, Robin is a computer whiz. She'd be a tremendous asset to her sister's company. I've watched her take an expensive, highly-complex computer apart, identify and replace a broken component, and reassemble the beast in less time than it takes me to type this page.

Robin said Ellen Connes, who had been overseeing medications and personal services, would replace her as director, reporting to Dennis Scalpone. Dennis was presently director of The Place at Tanque Verde and would divide his managerial duties between the two houses, both of which were owned by National Health Investors, Inc.

Next, Robin hit me with another bombshell. She and Lisa Jaramillo, her supervisor, joined forces to convince me I should place Maxine in hospice. To me, hospice is the last resort for anyone with a life-limiting illness. I hated the word "terminal," as it applied to hospice care.

After much discussion, I acquiesced and accepted Dr. Kentro's recommendation, VistaCare Hospice. Ruth Cook, a longtime registered nurse, was named VistaCare's team leader for Maxine. While at times I was a bit impatient with Ruth and her associates, I later realized they were actually doing more for Maxine than they did for some of their other patients. And I've since found the historic origins of hospice most fascinating.

Beginning in Europe in the 12th century, hospices provided lodging and care for weary pilgrims, the ill and the poor. In 1967, Dr. Cicely Saunders, founder of the modern hospice movement, established St. Christopher's Hospice in London, England. Eventually hospices and the hospice philosophy, which places both patients and their loved ones at the center of a model of holistic care, spread to America.

Hospice care does not replace the work of staff at facilities such as The Place. Instead, it's actually an extension of residence care. It's concerned with the physical, social, spiritual, and emotional comfort of patients rather than cure. Care is provided by a team of skilled hospice professionals and volunteers. In 1982, Medicare established the hospice benefit, expanding the growth and availability of hospice services throughout the United States. It even paid for Maxine's wheelchair and other medical equipment.

Members of VistaCare's team visited The Place several times a week to bathe, feed and examine Maxine. They worked closely with residence caregivers and nurses and maintained records of her vital statistics, general physical condition, and progress of her disease. They also monitored me and made suggestions if they thought I was doing something detrimental. Example: In talking to Maxine, I'd stress how much I "needed" her. Ruth Cook said that in Maxine's confused mind, she might think she'd done something wrong and begin worrying about it.

But a memorable incident occurred in April that confirmed what I'd long suspected. There were times when Max's instant reaction to a specific situation indicated that the mind had functioned as if she were in full command of all her faculties. It happened on Robin's last day at The Place.

I was sitting with Maxine in the TV room when an attractive young lady named Liz, whose two parents were also residents of The Place, walked up. She put her arm around me and said, "Jim, what are we going to do without Robin, she was so supportive of both of us?" I took her arm and said, "Well, Liz, we'll just have to support each other!"

Max observed and heard this, which she may have interpreted as a demonstration of mutual affection, judging from the expression on her face. With sparks in her eyes, she looked first at Liz, then me, and exclaimed, "Not good!" Robin happened by at that moment. She got down on her knees in front of Max and asked, "Is Jim Greenwood your special man?" Max: "Yes!"

In recent weeks I'd considered moving Maxine to a residence closer to home, strictly as a matter of convenience. There were three in Green Valley at the time, four if you count La Posada's small Alzheimer's unit in its healthcare building. (La Posada now has an upscale facility exclusively for Alzheimer's.) Prestige, an assisted living apartment house with a wing for demented residents, was a possibility. But after interviews with the director and his head nurse, I ruled it out.

Next my friend Adria Ackerman, a supervising nurse at Holy Cross Hospital in Nogales, Arizona, escorted me on a tour of Silver Springs and Santa Rita Care Center, also in Green Valley. Adria knew the staff at both places and vouched for their qualifications. Before I could reach a decision, however, it became obvious that Maxine's disease had progressed to the point where a change of venue was both unwise and impractical.

In May, we enjoyed a Mother's Day visit from my daughter Roxie, granddaughter Heather and her husband Scott Rider, and our great granddaughter Ashley Grace. Dinner places had been set for us in the library and the meal was delicious. I fed Max, who ate much of her pureed turkey and gravy, broccoli, two glasses of lemonade and a generous helping of ice cream. We wished Max a Happy Mother's Day, and she said, "That's why we're here!"

During the next few weeks, Max continued to eat fairly well, but she seemed more tired and spent quite a bit of time on her bed, in the mornings, as well as afternoons. I'd lie beside her and reminisce about our travels -- cruising along the Mexican Riviera, driving down the Florida Keys, searching for artifacts on the Custer battlefield in Montana. She winced when I mentioned our aborted sailing venture on Chesapeake Bay.

We'd rented an almost new 35-foot Brewster sloop with another couple for a relaxing weekend of sailing. First, the girls had emerged from the galley, slightly green, and said if we fellows wanted any breakfast, we had to fix it ourselves. Next the wind died down and we were becalmed in the shipping lane. We started the auxiliary engine and snapped the drive shaft. Twelve hours later, "Little Toot," a small tug from the marina, rescued us. Max said at the time she'd never again set foot on a sailboat.

I told Max I had another speech to deliver and that I'd seek her help, as always, in drafting it. I thought I'd start it by saying, "I learned long ago that there are three things in life you should never do: Never climb a ladder leaning toward you, never kiss a girl leaning away from you, and never talk to an audience that may know more about the subject than you do." Then I said, "I love you Max." And she said, "I love you too."

Max was grinding her teeth again. Hospice nurses recommended some sort of medication to relieve her toothaches. But Dr. Kentro opposed prescribing anything at this time as it might over sedate her. Later he prescribed Risperdal, a fairly strong sedative. I told Ruth Cook that Max didn't handle such a potent drug very well. For now, we won't use it.

VistaCare's Chaplain Keith Huffman visited Max and said a prayer for both of us. He noticed that I was quite anxious over Maxine's languid behavior, even though I had tried to prepare myself for the expected changes in her physical dimension. As he departed, the chaplain said, "Now Maxine, you take good care of Jim." She grinned.

The hospice's compassionate medical expertise supports peace in the body, which in turn invites spiritual and emotional peace, and release. They kept telling me dying is safe, that body, mind, and spirit undergo a harmless transformation. (Keep that in mind when you think of your own mortality.) And I told myself over and over again that only the body dies -- love does not.

Helene of VistaCare, probably exposed to death or near death almost every working day, had seen a dramatic decline in Maxine's physical condition, and an elevation in my denial. She may have thought I was hoping and praying for some sort of divine intervention that would make things right again. Helene sat me down and quietly said, "Face it, Jim, Maxine is dying."

Naturally, when the body weakens, it requires more care. As all contact with the rhythms of the physical world is lost, sleep is irregular and more frequent. (This sleep may actually be a time of life review and inner preparation.) It was up to me, the hospice team and the house staff to make sure Maxine was comfortable and free of any pain as she began her passage across the great divide. Still, my love for Max was so deep and strong I found it almost impossible to accept reality.

I informed my girls that they should make plans to visit once more while Maxine could sit up and enjoy them. Vivienne and her daughter Michele came over and spent an afternoon with us. Maxine was seated in the TV room and seemed to be very happy in the company of daughter and granddaughter. When Max showed signs of getting sleepy, we wheeled her back to 807.

All through July, Max averaged less than 50 percent of her meals, not including her supplement, which she relished. Her accelerated downhill slide started in August. Watching her slip away like that tore at my heartstrings; I felt so helpless. Jackie, a hospice volunteer, reported that Max was now resisting dinner, her main meal. Jackie also was unable to seat Max on the shower chair, so she gave her a bed-bath instead. The hospice bathing was in addition to the weekly showers that staff caregivers gave Max.

By mid-August, Max was spending more time in bed, and I was spending more time at her side. She even dozed off at the dining room table. I had to hold her head up, but she kept her mouth closed. It was all we could do to get Max to drink anything, including her supplement. I'm sure she was dehydrating.

Ruth Cook put a hold on two medications the hospice doctor had prescribed -- Clonazepam and Zyprexa -- because she felt Max was unable to tolerate either one, much less both. By now Maxine's vital signs were being taken at periodic intervals day and night. Her blood pressure, pulse and respiratory readings varied widely between highs and lows. She weighed 104 pounds August 8 and 98 on August 15, a loss of six pounds in one week.

Caregivers were told that if Maxine wanted to eat, fine. But don't force her. She was having more diffficulty swallowing, which seemed to get worse each succeeding day. In the following week, Max would lose another two pounds, putting her weight at 96 -- the lowest since she was a young teenager.

Whether morning or afternoon, I'd lay down with my precious and tell her more stories. One morning, I told her I'd spent an hour the previous night outdoors, viewing the bewildering array of countless millions of stars. It was a very clear night, just right for star gazing. I said, "It reminded me of your abiding interest in astronomy, Maxine. You took a course in it at the University of Illinois, where you majored in journalism, and you got an A."

I also told Max she still had her class textbook, *Introduction to Astronomy*, the only U of I textbook she had saved all these years. It was written by her professor, Robert A. Baker. "I wonder what Professor Baker would say," I said to Max, "if he knew a star had been named for you." She just smiled, then took my hand and kissed it.

Max ate a little better on August 16. The next day Glenna had to move Max around some to position her properly on the toilet seat. Max, disturbed by all the jostling, said, "Let's not go there." Before returning Max to her bed, Glenna swabbed her teeth with a special sponge stick and said, "There, Maxine, isn't that better?" Max: "It looks good."

On August 18, Ruth Cook noticed a rash and some swelling around one of Maxine's toes. She suggested the caregivers stop using T.E.D. hose on Max for at least a week. Ruth also asked Rosie to inform Doctors Kentro and Wessel, Maxine's podiatrist. The next day Maxine consumed 75 percent of her breakfast, half of her dinner and just a few bites of supper. She also refused to drink her supplement, a rare occurrence.

Dennis Scalpone called me early in the morning of August 20 to let me know that Max had apparently fallen out of her wheelchair while attempting to stand up. (Her chair featured a special cushion for comfort, but its design begged an inadvertent slip.) Andy Colussy, Dr. Kentro's nurse, examined Max and found nothing more serious than a bump on the nose and a two-inch red streak on the right abdomen. Andy also told us Maxine's stool was black with traces of blood. And the way her eyes looked, she must have had another TIA.

VistaCare Hospice had recently installed bedrails on both sides of Maxine's bed to prevent her from falling out. The hospice also furnished a new "egg crate" mattress to minimize her chances for acquiring bedsores during a prolonged stay in bed; two more freebies, thanks to Medicare.

The next few days were extremely hard, especially after Ruth told me Maxine's legs were swelling and colorizing. The condition is something like edema, but it's called mottle. It's caused by a lack of oxygen, which impedes the circulation of blood in the lower extremeties. When Ruth said it was a sign the end was near, I nearly collapsed. I had to steel myself again as I watched Max go through the early stage of withdrawal, a sharply declining appetite, and thirst.

I told myself a different energy may sustain Max now, a different kind of nourishment was needed -- one of "being with" rather than "doing for." VistaCare's team had one main message for me: I must trust that my loving presence was now my greatest gift to Maxine. Still, my grief intensified as the whole natural process of dying became very real.

My stepdaughter Marquita Brown, her husband Loren, and my brother-in-law Don Gladding and his wife Nell, arrived on August 23 for a short visit. Loren sat down on the bed with Max and said a prayer. Marquita also sat on the bed and talked to her. She then kissed her, misty-eyed. Finally, the Browns and Gladdings had to leave for their respective homes in Yorba Linda, California, and Sun City West near Phoenix. They would never see Maxine again.

Helene of VistaCare confirmed that Max was indeed dehydrated, but my precious still refused to drink anything. Debbie, also of hospice, said if other meds, such as Tylenol, failed to relieve any pain, VistaCare would prescribe morphine. On Ausust 25, Maxine was more restless on her bed than usual and appeared to have a severe pain in the intestinal area (her urine was dark and concentrated). Ruth ordered morphine drops for immediate delivery.

For some unknown reason, the pharmacy sent morphine in syrup form, but quickly replaced it with drops when they learned of their mistake. Unfortunately, Gina had already given Max a half-teaspoon full of the syrup sedative by the time Ruth became aware of the mixup. Ruth instructed Gina on the proper dosage using an eyedropper. The administration of morphine, incidentally, relieved Max of her pain almost instantly.

Chaplain Huffman came to 807, sat on the edge of Maxine's bed and said another prayer for the two of us. Max had been in and out of a deep sleep, but was awake at the time of the chaplain's visit and listened intently. As the chaplain got up to leave, he again said, "Now Maxine, you take good care of Jim." Max smiled.

Tuesday, August 26, and Wednesday, August 27, 2003, I spent most of the day and all night with Maxine. Debbie said they were able to feed Max a little food and part of her supplement early on Tuesday. Andy Colussy came back to the apartment and took Maxine's vitals again. All readings were unusually high. Her breathing was labored. Andy also commented on Max's legs, mottling had really taken hold, and the pronounced tremor in her hands. Even though she slept most of the day, I was beside her, talking about us.

At 4:45 p.m., I told Gina I'd be staying overnight with my precious. Call it a premonition, intuition, or whatever, I simply knew I had to be there with her.

It was pouring rain outside and by the time I reached the car I was soaking wet. I raced home through one of the worst thunderstorms of the monsoon season, got my overnight case and returned to Max in 65 minutes.

As I crawled in bed beside her, I remembered what Ruth Cook had told me. According to medical science, hearing is the last sense to go after all other systems of the body close down. So I held Maxine's hand in mine and talked. She had been looking up at the ceiling, now she turned her head and focused her pretty blue eyes on me.

It was uncanny, but Maxine actually looked much younger than she did earlier in the day. In fact, her face radiated a bright, angelic aura that made her more beautiful than ever. I squeeze her hand as I kissed her, then recited that popular children's bedtime prayer several times:

> *Now I lay me down to sleep,*
> *I pray the Lord my soul to keep.*
> *If I should die before I wake,*
> *I pray the Lord my soul to take.*

Gina took Maxine's vitals at 9:30 p.m. -- blood pressure 90 over 62, pulse 112 and temperature 101.7. She also ordered a hospice oral suction device to remove any excess saliva that might accumulate in Maxine's mouth. Max closed her eyes intermittently, but when open she looked directly at me.

Gina said that even when Maxine's eyes were closed and she appeared to be sleeping, she was very much aware that I was with her. Whenever I got up to go to the bathroom, Max's breathing became faster, according to Gina. And when I came back and got in bed, her breathing became more relaxed.

Michele and Kelly (3rd shift) came on duty at 11 p.m. After midnight, they checked on us every 30 minutes. As long as I talked to her, Max kept looking at me. Shortly after the 2:30 a.m. check I dozed off briefly. I awoke abruptly at 3. Maxine's head was turned toward me. Her eyes and mouth were open and her breathing had stopped. Tears welled up in my eyes as I called Michele and Kelly. They came right in and saw that Maxine's long struggle with Alzheimer's disease was over. She had departed this troubled planet peacefully and with grace and dignity.

The girls withdrew from the apartment to give me a few minutes alone with my precious. I was still lying beside her and holding her hand. There were so many things I wanted to say, but all I could manage was: I love you, I love you, I love you Maxine. And I tried holding back the tears, but just couldn't. Max wouldn't like it if she saw me crying.

I let go of her hand and cupped her face between my palms. Then I embraced her warmly, pulled her chin up tenderly, and kissed her once more on the lips. Finally, with fingers still trembling slightly, I reached over and gently closed her eyes for the last time.

EPILOGUE

*The transition from life can be every bit as profound,
intimate and precious as the miracle of birth.*

Ira Byock, M.D.

VistaCare Hospice was notified immediately and Cindy Powell, an RN, arrived within 20 minutes. She examined Maxine and officially verified her demise. She promptly informed Max's doctor, Tenney Kentro, and the Green Valley Mortuary where I had made arrangements in advance for both Maxine and me. Many years ago, we had decided on cremation, though at first Maxine had some doubts, saying, "But that's so final."

Max was transferred to Green Valley by Mike McCully of Southwest Mortuary Service. He was extremely caring as he removed her from Apartment 807 in The Place at Tucson. Meanwhile, Ellen Connes and members of her staff gathered in 807 to offer their condolences, and to tell me how much they thought of Maxine as a human being.

On August 28, my daughter Jeanne flew in from Georgia to help me with details and comfort me during the first few days of my grief. I didn't ask her to come, she just thought I needed someone near and dear who might ease the pain of my tremendous loss. Jeanne and my other girls, Roxanne and Karen, were very fond of their stepmother. And they had shown their affection in many ways.

On September 11, 2003, our 33rd wedding anniversary, I interred Maxine in the Columbarium at the Valley Presbyterian Church in Green Valley, Arizona. It was a private memorial service with Rev. John Dunham, associate pastor of the church, officiating. The only others present were Julee Dawson, a deputy director of the Arizona Aerospace Foundation, one of the last outsiders to see

Max, and Edward Ackerman, also a good friend.

The weekend before Maxine's 87th birthday (October 20, 2003), Marquita and Loren Brown held a celebration of life in their Yorba Linda home. Family and friends gathered for an afternoon of reminiscing about their more memorable experiences in the company of Maxine. Michael Donaldson, my nephew, joined me in representing the Greenwood side of the union. I recalled a number of amusing incidents in our life together, but when I came to the punch line, I'd choke up.

One member of our group mentioned the many hours of volunteer service Maxine devoted to various institutions, such as American Red Cross, Wichita Art Museum, and other worthy causes. I added the days she spent managing the office of Camp Tapawingo, a Virginia-based charitable facility for disadvantaged children. And who'd ever forget all her work for the American Association of University Women (she was an honorary life member), and that her bio appeared in the Marquis *Who's Who of American Women*.

Perhaps the most difficult piece of writing I've ever done was Maxine's obituary, even though I knew all the elements like the back of my hand. It was published in the *Green Valley News and Sun*, *Arizona Daily Star* and *The Wichita Eagle*. It also went out over the Internet, prompting friends and relatives in distant states to call or send their condolences.

The outpouring of genuine affection for Maxine touched my heart. Of all the cards and letters I received, and there were many, a very special one from longtime friend Wendy Dresang best described the impression Max left with everyone she met. Wendy wrote it to herself many years ago and found it tucked away in one of her address books. It's worth repeating here:

> *It is always a privilege to be in the presence of Maxine. She expresses a grace and strength that goes beyond words and actions. She is truly a good and beautiful person.*

I'll always be indebted to many people for their wonderful support during and after the most trying time of my life. I'm especially grateful for the love and concerns of my extended family -- my three daughters: Roxanne, Jeanne and Karen; and stepdaughters Yvonne, Marquita and Vivienne. They were an enormous help to me through the dark years of Maxine's dementia. I don't think I could have coped without knowing they were always there for me at anytime I might send up a distress signal.

My heartfeld thanks to Robin Henson and her staff at The Gardens and The

Place at Tucson for their compassion, sensitivity, and excellent care while Maxine was in residence in each respective home. And to Ruth Cook and her VistaCare Hospice team who did so much for Maxine and me during the last few months of her life.

I also owe a debt of gratitude to Jessie V. Pergrin, RN, PhD, for her helpful counsel over the years. A widely-recognized authority on Alzheimer's, Jessie unselfishly gives much of her time and energy to those whose loved ones are victims of this dreaded disease. She established and still leads Alzheimer's support groups in southern Arizona and plays a key role in other important programs aimed at providing technical and operational guidance to professional caregivers.

Following Maxine's interment, I became a member of the Church Columbarium Committee. One of my first duties as a member was to help select something inspirational for the Columbarium's open interior space. Upon the recommendation of the University of Arizona, we chose Lauri Slenning, a talented sculptress who does magnificent fine art in bronze, to submit a proposal. The result was an eight-foot bronze statue of eight doves flying into the heavens from a circular base titled Ascension. It adds a unique spiritual dimension within the Columbarium's sacred walls.

My grateful thanks to Bernie Freeman and Jeff Roley of the University of Illinois Foundation, and to the late Kim Rotzoll, dean of the U of I's College of Communications, for bringing Maxine's alma mater into her "home" through visitations and correspondence. When they discussed the University in front of Max, you could tell by her expression she understood much of what they were saying.

My thanks to Carol Barry Nelson of Type & Graphics for her typography and graphic design of this book. Carol, a highly-respected and skilled professional in her specialized field, has typed and edited most of my manuscripts and speeches ever since Maxine's disease made her incapable of doing so.

Very special thanks to worldy-wise Helen Johnson, who nursed me through several serious health issues and made me believe there could be life after death. Helen is a dear friend, an articulate conversationalist and an enjoyable companion whose advice on physical therapy -- and many other things as well -- is highly valued. She's a wonderful person.

And to the Alzheimer's Association, my sincere appreciation for the fine work it's doing. Perhaps it's not yet widely known, but the organization offers a free helpline with 24/7 assistance for patients, families, and caregivers. Calls are confidential, and the telephones are staffed by master's-level clinicians who can provide information about dementia, crisis assistance, caregiving and treatment options. The helpline (1-800-272-3900) answers more than 250,000 calls a year.

I'm still a supporter of the Association and especially of the Alzheimer's research it continues to fund. Of particular interest to me is the recent effort of the Alzheimer's Institute of Cal State Channel Islands, which may hold considerable promise. Cal State scientists are focused on chemically altering oils from plants such as ginger and ginko biloba and testing the extracts' ability to treat and prevent the disease. They note that many modern drugs and medicines are derived from plant sources and view plant oils as potential weapons against the scourge.

I haven't decided if a riskier approach to research is a proper way to go. Some scientists are tentatively exploring a handful of bold, sometimes invasive procedures -- from another vaccine attempt to gene therapy that requires brain injections. Yet some families battling the disease say they'd take the risk, even a drug with a 50 percent chance of death, if there were an equal opportunity for benefits.

For my beloved Maxine, however, her transition is complete. She's at peace now in a better place, leaving behind a battered world peppered with pockets of cruelty, conflict, and corruption. Maxine was adored and admired by many, and she is greatly missed. And in the not-too-distant future in the Columbarium niche next to hers, I will be reunited with my precious forevermore, just as it was meant to be.

Printed in the United States
48174LVS00002B/157-204

9 781587 366352